HAPPY, HEALTHY, AND FIT!

Whole Health Activities for Children Ages 4–8

Carolyn Luetje
Carol Quinn

illustrated by Shannon Quinn-Schneck

THE CENTER FOR APPLIED
RESEARCH IN EDUCATION
West Nyack, New York 10995

10 9 8 7 6 5 4 3 2 1

Library of Congress Cataloging-in-Publication Data

Luetje, Carolyn.
Happy, healthy, and fit! : whole health activities for children ages 4–8 / Carolyn Luetje and Carol Quinn ; illustrated by Shannon Quinn-Schneck.
p. cm.
Includes bibliographical references.
ISBN 0–87628–381–4
1. Health education (Elementary) 2. Education, Elementary--Activity programs. I. Quinn, Carol. II. Title.
LB1587.A3L84 1992
372.3′7–dc20 91–21634
CIP

THE CENTER FOR APPLIED
RESEARCH IN EDUCATION
BUSINESS & PROFESSIONAL DIVISION
A division of Simon & Schuster
West Nyack, New York 10995

Printed in the United States of America

We dedicate this book to

Jessica,
Emily,
and
Jacob

Sean
and
Megan

and all children everywhere

ABOUT THE AUTHORS

Carolyn Luetje received a Bachelor of Science degree from Iowa State University and an Early Childhood Certificate from the University of California, Los Angeles. She has been a preschool teacher since 1971.

Carol Quinn attended Los Angeles City College and El Camino College, Torrance, California. She has been a teacher in Child Development in the Los Angeles City Schools Children's Centers and a storyteller for the Torrance Public Library System.

Together the authors have written eight resource books for early childhood teachers.

ABOUT THIS BOOK

Happy, Healthy, and Fit! Whole Health Activities for Children Ages 4–8 is designed to help teachers of children in preschool through second grade introduce their students to the basics of good health. As the children participate in the activities in this book, they will also begin to understand ways in which they can take responsibility for their own health.

The activities in *Happy, Healthy, and Fit!* teach children about health in ways that will stimulate their interest and encourage their participation. Each of the eight sections of the book contains individual, small group, and whole class activities. In addition, there are many poems and action verses which will capture the children's interest as they learn.

An additional feature of this book is the inclusion of pages from which students can assemble individual "Here's to My Health" booklets. Each of these pages is marked with a distinctive bird logo for easy identification by both students and teachers. As students color pictures, record safety information, and keep personal health records, they will gain an appreciation of their own health and how to maintain it. The booklets will also give students a permanent record of what they have learned and enable them to share their knowledge of good health with their families.

Happy, Healthy, and Fit! can be used as a supplement to an existing health program, or as a guide for setting up and implementing a new health curriculum. The book is divided into eight sections, with each section covering an important aspect of good health:

- NUTRITION . . . The 11 activities in this section introduce students to a variety of nutritious foods, teach them about the four food groups, and encourage them to choose a well-balanced diet.
- RECIPES . . . 26 easy-to-prepare recipes are included that reinforce concepts of good nutrition, and help students practice food preparation techniques and safe use of kitchen equipment and appliances.
- HEALTH HABITS . . . This section includes 15 activities which teach students how to keep themselves healthy, establish good health routines, and become comfortable with health care professionals.
- FEELINGS AND SELF-ESTEEM . . . This section includes 18 activities that help students recognize, understand, and express their feelings. These activities also help each student develop a positive self-image.
- SAFETY . . . The 17 activities in this section introduce common safety rules and teach students how to respond safely to everyday and emergency situations.
- EXERCISE . . . The 30 activities in this section stress the importance of being physically fit, and encourage students to make exercise part of their daily routines.
- SUBSTANCE ABUSE PREVENTION . . . The seven activities in this section teach students to recognize harmful substances, and help them develop and practice techniques for refusing those substances. Research shows that the more health education students receive, the less likely they are to use alcohol and other drugs.

- GAMES AND DANCES . . . A variety of games and dances are included that reinforce concepts introduced in the other sections. The 44 games and dances also offer opportunities for students to interact socially, move and exercise their muscles and bodies, and participate in enjoyable activities together.

Happy, Healthy, and Fit! contains ready-to-use activity sheets for students to complete in conjunction with many of the activities. Teacher directions are included, explaining how and when to integrate each activity sheet with the corresponding activity. In addition, easy-to-understand student directions are printed on each activity sheet. Several sections contain games, puzzles, and other high-interest activities designed to capture students' attention and help them remember what they have learned. Review sheets are also provided that may be placed in learning centers or given to students for independent use. A "Resource List" is provided with titles of books, records, cassettes, and videotapes that supplement the activities and reinforce the concepts presented in all eight sections of the book.

Learned early, good health habits can have positive effects that last for a lifetime. By helping young children understand and practice ways to care for and protect their bodies, you can make an important difference in your students' health and lives!

Carolyn Luetje
Carol Quinn

HOW TO MAKE "HERE'S TO MY HEALTH" BOOKLETS

As the children in your class participate in the *Happy, Healthy, and Fit!* activities that follow, they will be learning how to care for their own health. Help students remember what they learn, and share it at home, by assembling individual "Here's to My Health" booklets.

Materials:

- copies of "Here's to My Health" booklet cover
- 9″ x 12″ construction paper
- crayons or colored markers
- yarn, fabric scraps, or other decorative materials
- glue
- hand mirrors or wall mirror
- file folder for each student
- stapler

Directions:

Distribute the "Here's to My Health" booklet covers. Have each student glue a cover to a sheet of construction paper. Then ask students to look in a mirror to see the color of their eyes, hair, and skin. Have each child color the face on the booklet cover to resemble himself or herself. Provide short pieces of yarn to glue on for hair, ribbon or fabric scraps for hair ribbons or bow ties, and other decorations. Give each child a file folder in which to put the finished booklet cover.

Point out the bird logo in the upper left corner of the "Here's to My Health" booklet cover. Explain that the bird is a symbol that will show students the pages to put in their booklets. Explain that each time they complete a page on which they see that symbol, they should add that page to their file folders. When all of the pages marked with the bird logo have been completed, help students stack their papers with the "Here's to My Health" booklet cover on top. Staple through each student's stack of papers, along the left side, to complete the booklets.

The following pages should go into the "Here's to My Health" booklets:

- Four food group pictures (activity sheets 1–1A through 1–1D
- Four picture recipes (activity sheets 2–22A, 2–23A, 2–25A, and 2–26A)
- Toothbrushing Chart (activity sheet 3–1A)
- Watch Me Grow! Chart (activity sheet 3–12A)
- All About Me (activity sheet 4–12B)
- Emergency Number (activity sheet 5–15A)
- Exercise Chart (activity sheet 6–3B)
- Substance Abuse Game Sheet (activity sheet 7–3A)

Encourage students to take their completed "Here's to My Health" booklets home to share with their families. Suggest that they show the booklet pages to family members, and explain what they have learned about staying healthy.

CONTENTS

3 = HEALTH HABITS • 73

4 = FEELINGS AND SELF-ESTEEM • 111

5 = SAFETY • 145

6 = EXERCISE • 189

7 = SUBSTANCE ABUSE PREVENTION • 231

8 = GAMES AND DANCES • 253

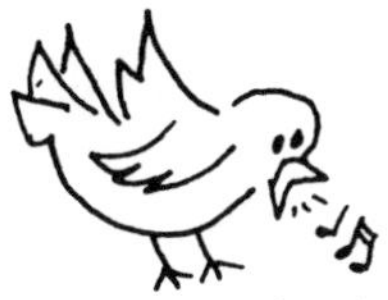

"Here's to My Health"

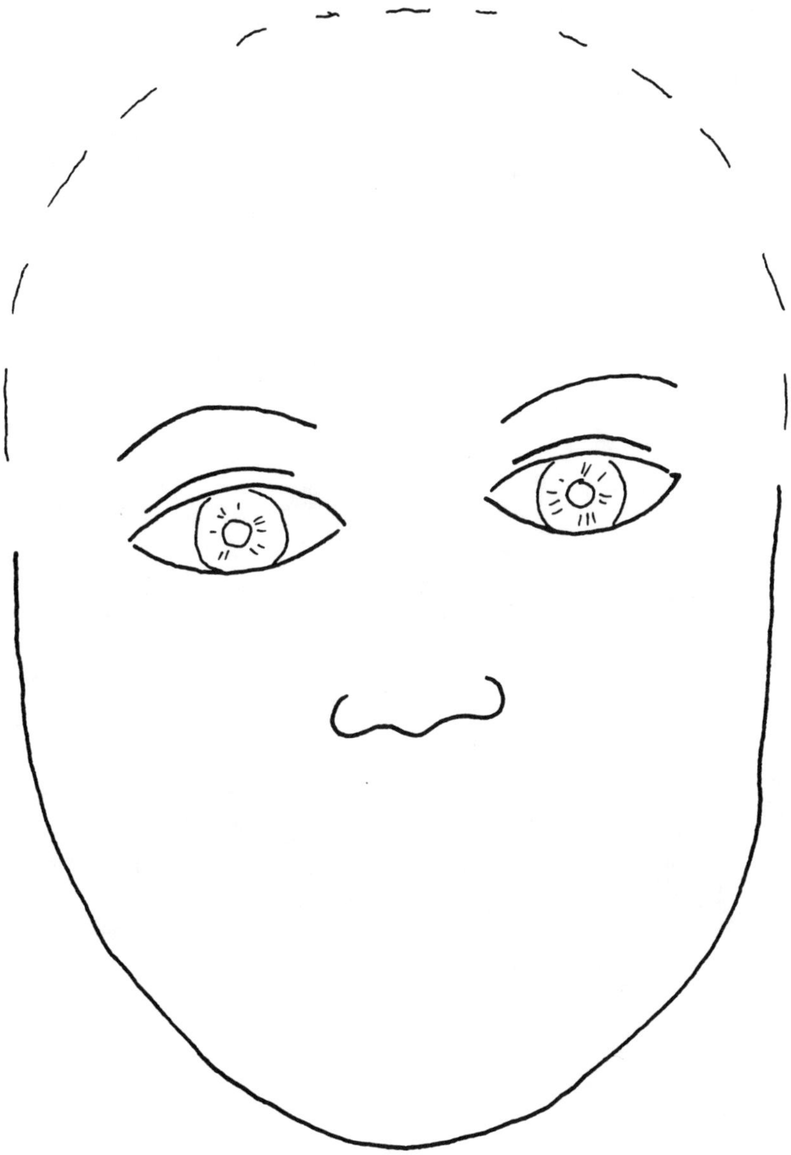

Name ______________________________

1 — NUTRITION

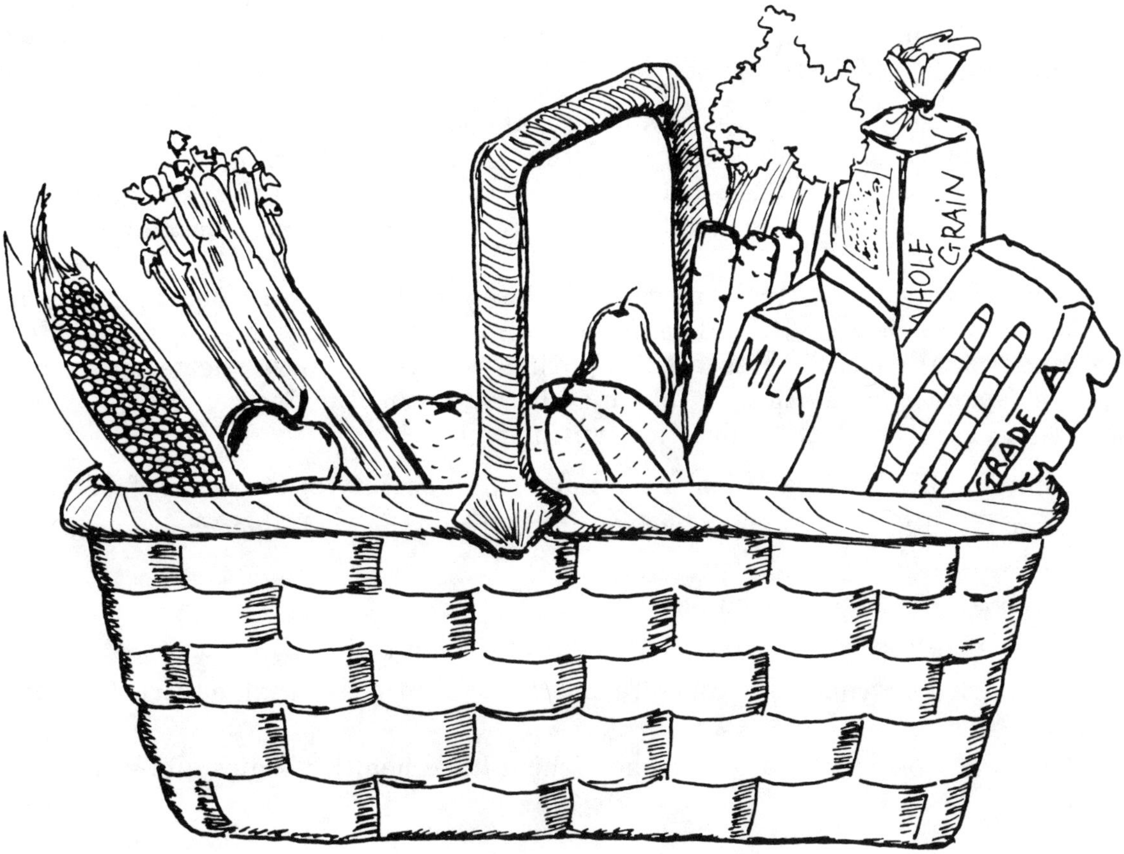

Teaching young children about good nutrition can influence their eating habits and their health as they get older. If children learn to choose healthy, nutritious foods at a young age, they will be more likely to make healthy choices in the years to come.

Medical and nutrition researchers report that:

- overweight children as young as five or six years old can have elevated blood pressure;
- dietary habits formed in children's early years can influence their risk of heart disease when they become adults;
- about 20 percent of 12,000 children in one study had cholesterol levels above 200;
- children who make their own choices about snacks tend to select those that are high in fat and sugar.

Most four- to eight-year-olds are not able to make judgments about which foods are high in cholesterol, fat, sodium, or sugar. However, they can learn which foods are nutritious and which are not; they can learn to eat more fish, poultry, fruits, vegetables, and grains; and they can learn to choose fresh fruit, vegetables, and whole grain products instead of high-calorie sugary snacks.

The activities which follow will introduce children to simple nutritional concepts and help them understand the basics of a well-balanced diet. Several review sheets are included which reinforce nutritional concepts presented in earlier activities. These sheets may be used for review, as independent activities, or they may be placed in learning centers.

The activities in the Nutrition section will help students:

- become familiar with and learn the names of a variety of nutritious foods;
- become familiar with the four food groups and how the foods in each group contribute to good health;
- sort foods into the four food groups;
- learn to chose nutritious foods for meals and snacks;
- distinguish between foods that are nutritious and those that have little nutritional value;
- understand that nutritious foods help them have healthy bodies and minds.

1–1 EAT RIGHT EVERY DAY

Begin your study of nutrition by introducing students to the four food groups.

Materials:

copies of activity sheets 1–1A, 1–1B, 1–1C, and 1–1D
tagboard, approximately 2′ x 3′
marker
crayons
glue

Preparation:

1. Make a food group poster by writing the title EAT RIGHT EVERY DAY at the top of the tagboard. Draw lines to divide the tagboard into four sections, each approximately 12″ x 18″.
2. Glue a food group picture in each section. You may wish to have students color the food pictures.
3. Display the poster at the children's eye level.

Directions:

Point out the EAT RIGHT EVERY DAY poster and read the captions aloud. Help students identify each of the foods in the food group pictures.

Ask students to name and point out foods they have eaten today or yesterday. Then have them point out their favorite foods. Help students understand that our bodies are like machines and that in order to operate they need the right kind of fuel. Explain that food is fuel for our bodies.

Discuss the importance of eating foods from the four food groups each day. Talk about other foods, such as chips, doughnuts, or candy that have little nutritional value. Help students understand that it is all right to eat those foods once in a while.

Distribute a set of the food group activity sheets to each student. Have students color the pictures and then add the sheets to their "Here's to My Health" booklet file folders.

1–2 FUN-WITH-FOOD GAMES

Help students learn about nutrition while having fun with the following games. Have students complete their food group activity sheets 1–1A through 1–1D before playing the games. Then review the food groups with students and discuss how each type of food helps our bodies grow strong and healthy.

Directions:

Several of the "Fun With Food" games require food cards. Make food cards by reproducing the Food Pictures pages 1–2A and 1–2B. Cut both pages apart to make 24 individual pictures. Glue each food picture to an index card or a 3″ construction paper square. You may wish to have students color the food pictures. Cover the food cards with clear self-adhesive vinyl to make them more durable.

PICK-A-PICTURE

Number of Players:

4–6

Material:

food cards (see directions)

How to Play:

Have all the players sit in a circle on the floor. Spread the food cards face down in the middle of the circle.

Have players take turns picking a food card, naming the food, and giving a "thumbs up" signal for a healthy food or a "thumbs down" signal for an unhealthy food.

FISH FOR FOOD

Number of Players:

2–4

Materials:

food cards (see directions)
small paper clips
18″ dowel
small magnet
36″ piece of string

Preparation:

1. Attach a paper clip to each food card.
2. Make a fishing pole by tying one end of the string around the magnet. Tie the other end of the string around the end of the dowel.

How to Play:

Spread the food cards face up on the floor. Have players take turns "fishing" for healthy foods, naming the foods they "catch," and naming the food groups to which they belong. If players catch foods that are not healthy, they should "throw them back," and try again.

BAG THE GROCERIES

Number of Players:

1–2

Materials:

food cards (see directions)
Food Group activity sheets 1–1A through 1–1D
crayons
plastic play foods
five large grocery bags or boxes
tape or stapler
empty food containers

Preparation:

1. Ask students to bring in a variety of empty food containers.
2. Reproduce one set of Food Group activity sheets. You may wish to have students color the pictures.
3. Tape or staple a food group picture to each of four bags or boxes. Write "Once in a While" on the fifth bag or box.

How to Play:

Place the grocery bags or boxes on a table. Spread out the food cards, plastic play foods, and empty food containers.

Have players sort the items into the bags or boxes according to food groups. Foods that are not healthy and nutritious should be put in the bag or box labeled "Once in a While."

GUESS WHAT'S GONE

Number of Players:

whole class

Materials:

tray
real foods, plastic play foods, or empty food containers

How to Play:

Put a selection of foods from the Milk Group on a tray. Have students look at the tray for about a minute, and then ask them to close their eyes. Remove one or two foods from the tray. Have students open their eyes, look at the tray, and name what's missing. Repeat with foods from other food groups.

NAME WHAT'S NEW

Number of Players:

whole class

Materials:

tray
real foods, plastic play foods, or empty food containers

How to Play:

Put the foods you removed in the "Guess What's Gone" game back on the tray. Have students look at the tray for about a minute, and then ask them to close their eyes. Add several new foods to the tray. Have students open their eyes, look at the tray, and name the foods you have added.

ALPHABET ANSWERS

Number of Players:

whole class

How to Play:

Ask the students to name as many nutritious foods as they can. Begin with A and continue through the alphabet, having students name a food that begins with each letter. If no one can think of an answer for a letter, have them make up the name of a food, draw a picture of it, and share it with the class. Display the pictures on the bulletin board.

Possible Foods:

A–apple, asparagus, apricot
B–banana, bean, beet, bread
C–carrot, cantaloupe, corn, cheese, chicken
D–date
E–eggs, eggplant
F–fish, figs
G–grapes, grapefruit
H–ham
I–ice cream
J–jicama, juice
K–kale, kohlrabi
L–lemons, limes, lettuce
M–milk, muffins, meat, macaroni
N–noodles, nuts, nectarines
O–oranges, onions, okra, oatmeal
P–potatoes, peaches, pears, peas, peanut butter
Q–make up the name of a food
R–rhubarb, rice, raisins, radishes, raspberries
S–spinach, spaghetti, squash, strawberries, shrimp
T–tomatoes, turkey, tuna, tangerines, turnips
U–make up the name of a food
V–make up the name of a food
W–watermelon, watercress
X–make up the name of a food
Y–yams, yogurt
Z–zucchini

FOOD HUNT

Number of Players:

whole class

Materials:

food cards (see directions)
chalk

Preparation:

1. Chalk five large circles on the floor.
2. Chalk the name of a food group near the outer edge of each circle. Label the fifth circle "Once in a While."

How to Play:

Point out the circles and read the names of the food groups aloud. Have students close their eyes while you hide the food cards in the room. When all the cards are hidden, ask each student to find one picture, and then sit in the circle labeled with the food group to which that food belongs. After everyone is sitting, have the students hold up their pictures one circle at a time. Ask each student to name the food and the food circle.

MAKE-A-MATCH

Number of Players:

2–4

Materials:

2 sets of food cards (see directions)

Preparation:

1. Remove the food cards showing the candy bar, cake, ice cream cone, french fries, doughnuts, and bag of chips for this game.

How to Play:

Have all the players sit in a circle on the floor. Mix all 36 food cards and spread them face down in the middle of the circle.

Have players take turns turning over two food cards at a time. If the pictures match, the player names the food and the food group to which it belongs, and keeps the pair of cards. If the cards do not match, the player places them face down on the floor again. Then the next player takes a turn. The game continues until all 18 pairs of pictures are matched.

FOOD LOTTO

Number of Players:

5

Materials:

2 identical sets of 36 food stickers (available from educational supply stores)
4 copies of Food Lotto Game Card 1–2C
clear self-adhesive vinyl (optional)
tagboard
scissors

Preparation:

1. Using one set of food stickers, attach a sticker to each section on the game cards. Make each game card different.
2. Cut the tagboard into 36 small cards, 2″ square.
3. Attach the other set of stickers to the small game cards.
4. You may wish to cover the game cards and the small cards with clear self-adhesive vinyl to make them more durable.

How to Play:

Designate one student as the leader and the other four as players. Have the leader gather all the small cards, mix them, and put them face down in a pile. Have each player choose a game card.

Have the leader show a small card to the players. The players look at their game cards to see if they have the same picture. Whoever has the picture names the food, takes the picture, and covers the matching picture on his or her game card. The first player to cover all nine pictures is the winner.

1–3 FOOD GROUP FESTIVAL

Plan a parade to celebrate healthy eating.

Materials:

- construction paper
- crayons or markers
- glue
- old magazines
- scissors

Directions:

Review the four food groups with students and discuss how foods in each group contribute to good health:

Milk Group: these foods help teeth and bones grow strong.

Meat Group: these foods build bones, muscles, and blood.

Fruit and Vegetable Group: these foods keep you healthy and heal cuts and bruises.

Bread and Cereal Group: these foods give you energy.

Divide students into four groups and assign each group to represent one of the four food groups. Have students make signs, using the materials above, that show foods from their food group.

Read the poem aloud and help each group learn their verse. Have the whole class learn the last verse.

Organize students in order by group (milk, meat, fruits and vegetables, breads and cereals). Then have students march around the room, with each group chanting its verse in turn and holding up its signs. Have all four groups chant the last verse together.

Milk:

Take three from the milk group
That's what we like to shout.
From milk, cheese, or yogurt
Pick three servings out.

Meat:

Take two from the meat group.
That's what we like to say,
Meat, poultry, fish or eggs
Take two servings each day.

Fruits and Vegetables:
Four from fruits or vegetables
That's what we like to call.
Oranges, carrots and lots more
Take four from them all.

Breads and Cereals:
Take four from breads and cereals
That's what we suggest.
Whole grains, rice and pastas
Four from these are best.

All:
Think of three, two, four, four
They're numbers we should know.
They add up to good nutrition
To help our bodies grow.

1–4 WONDERFUL WINDOW GARDEN

Here's a way to "sprout" fruits and vegetables in the classroom all year around.

Materials:

fruit and vegetable patterns 1–4A through 1–4D
construction paper (orange, brown, red, yellow, green)
tissue paper
(orange, brown, red, yellow)
glue
yarn
transparent tape
stapler
scissors

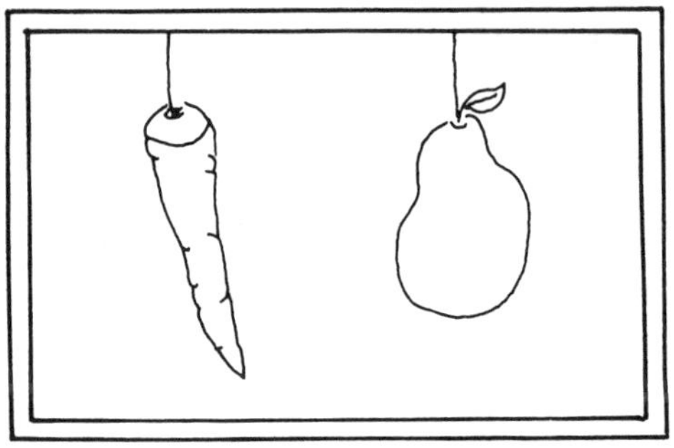

Preparation:

1. Trace the fruit and vegetable patterns onto construction paper, using the following colors: carrot–orange; onion–brown; apple–red; pear–yellow.
2. Cut out and discard the center section, leaving a paper outline of each fruit and vegetable.
3. Cut tissue paper, in the colors listed above, into 6″ x 8″ rectangles.

Older students may be able to do the above steps independently.

Directions:

Have each student choose a paper fruit or vegetable outline, spread glue along its edges, and lay a matching tissue paper rectangle on the glue. When the glue is dry, have the student trim away the excess tissue paper.

Next, have students cut out green construction paper leaves and glue them to the tops of the fruits or vegetables. Then help them staple on yarn loops for hanging. Help students tape their fruits and vegetables to a classroom window to make a "Wonderful Window Garden." Discuss with students the importance of eating a variety of fruits and vegetables every day.

1–5 FOOD MOBILE

Make mobiles to help students remember to eat four servings of fruits and vegetables every day.

Materials:

wire coat hangers
construction paper
string or yarn
cardboard
crayons or markers
scissors
glue
paper punch

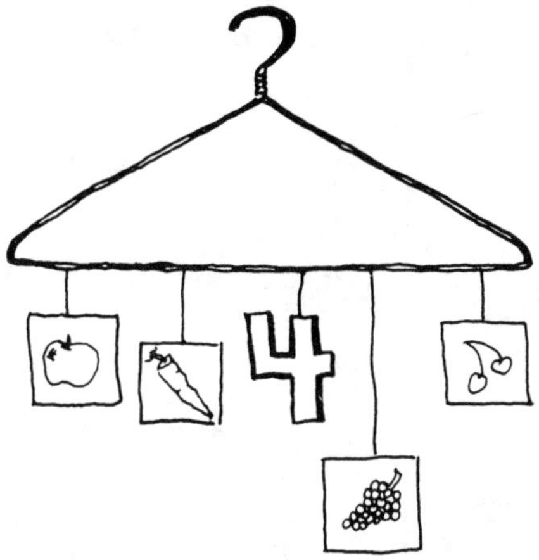

Preparation:

1. Cut a cardboard number 4 for each student, and punch a hole at the top.
2. Cut four 4″ squares of cardboard for each student.

Directions:

Have each student draw small pictures of four fruits and vegetables, and then cut them out and glue them to cardboard squares. Then have students punch a hole at the top of each picture and suspend it with string from the bottom of the coat hanger, making the strings different lengths so the pictures hang at different levels. (Younger students may need help with this step.) Have each student also hang the cardboard 4 from the coat hanger.

Encourage students to hang their mobiles at home as a reminder to eat four servings of fruits and vegetables every day.

1–6 LET'S EAT OUT

A make-believe restaurant can be the setting for choosing and learning about nutritious foods.

Materials:

construction paper
crayons or markers
scissors
old magazines
drawing paper
glue
food cards (see activity 1–2)
EAT RIGHT EVERY DAY poster (see activity 1–1)
table and chairs
paper plates and napkins
plastic knives, forks, spoons
plastic play foods
play money

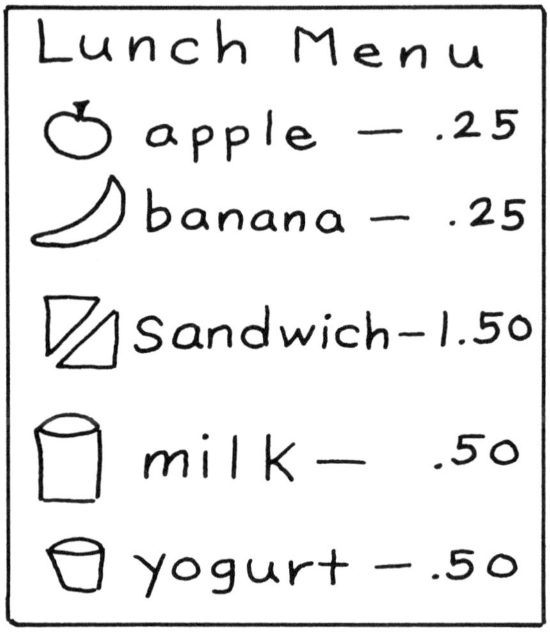

Preparation:

1. Write the words *Breakfast Menu* at the top of one sheet of construction paper, *Lunch Menu* at the top of the second sheet, and *Dinner Menu* on the third.
2. Arrange several chairs around a small table to resemble a restaurant setting.
3. Display the EAT RIGHT EVERY DAY poster nearby.

Directions:

Show the menus to the students and explain that menus show restaurant customers what foods are available. Have students draw small food pictures, or cut food pictures from magazines, and glue the pictures along the left side of the menus. Help students write the name of each food and its price. (See illustration.)

Have students set the table with paper napkins and plastic knives, forks, and spoons. Invite several students to be restaurant customers while one or two others are servers. Encourage the customers to order meals that include foods from each of the four food groups. Suggest that they look at the EAT RIGHT EVERY DAY poster to help them remember foods in each group. Have the servers fill the orders by placing plastic play foods or food cards on paper plates and serving them to the customers. After they "eat," have customers pay for their meals with play money.

1–7 THE FANTASY FRUIT TREE

What fun it would be to grow a fantasy fruit tree!

Materials:

butcher paper
crayons or markers
a variety of fresh or canned fruits
white construction paper
scissors

Preparation:

Draw and cut out the outline of a large tree on butcher paper.

Directions:

Let the students color the tree and draw branches on it. Pin the tree on a wall so that everyone can reach its branches.

Have the students draw, cut out, and color a variety of fruits on construction paper.

Read Verse 1 of the poem aloud. Ask students to chant the verse as each child pins a fruit on the tree. After all the fruits are on the tree, have students name them.

After the discussion, read Verse 2 aloud. Have students chant it as each child picks a fruit off the tree. Serve samples of fruits that might grow on a "Fantasy Fruit Tree."

Verse 1:

Fantasy fruit tree
Growing in the sun
With fabulous fruits
Showing one by one.

Verse 2:

Fantasy fruit tree
Picking time's near
With fabulous tastes
For everyone here.

1–8 VEGGIE VERSES

Encourage students to eat vegetables by reading these veggie riddles aloud.

Materials:

copies of Veggie Verses activity sheet 1–8A
crayons

Directions:

Read each verse aloud to the students. After each riddle, give them time to guess the name of the vegetable and draw a picture of it on the Veggie Verses activity sheet 1–8A. Then have students compare to see if they drew the same vegetables.

1. I have a lot of eyes
   But I can't see you know.
   Underneath the ground
   Is how I grow.
   (potato)

2. Look-alike green beads
   Together in a pod
   Growing on a vine
   Up above the sod.
   (peas)

3. Yellow kernels in a row.
   Green husks all around.
   Long ears on tall stalks
   Grow high off the ground.
   (corn)

4. Green tops above the soil,
   Orange down below.
   These two pretty colors
   Are what I show.
   (carrots)

1–9 A GLASS GARDEN

Alfalfa sprouts are a delicious and pretty way to decorate sandwiches, soups, and salads. Help students grow their own sprouts in a glass garden.

Materials:

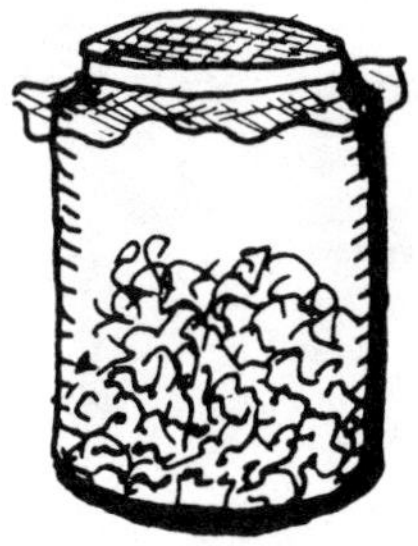

1 Tbsp. alfalfa seeds, available from health food stores
large wide-mouth glass jar with lid
water
fine cheesecloth, enough to cover jar mouth
rubber band

Directions:

Let students help put the alfalfa seeds into the jar, fill the jar with water, and put the cheesecloth over the jar opening, securing it with the rubber band. Let the seeds soak overnight.

The next morning, drain the water from the jar, but do not remove the cheesecloth. Ask a student to put fresh water in the jar. Drain all the water again. Put the jar on its side in a dark cupboard.

In the afternoon, rinse the seeds again and drain well. Shake the seeds gently to separate. Put the jar back on its side in the cupboard.

Have students help rinse and drain the sprouts twice a day for three or four days until small leaves appear. Remove the cheesecloth and put the lid on the jar. Store the sprouts in a tightly closed jar in the refrigerator. Let students add the sprouts to sandwiches, soups, and salads. One tablespoon of seeds makes two cups of sprouts.

1–10 SETTING THE TABLE

Help students learn to set the table properly.

Materials:

sponges cut into circles, triangles, or other shapes
shallow trays
tempera paint
newspapers
copies of Place Mat activity sheet 1–10A
plastic knives, forks, and spoons
paper plates, cups, and napkins
flowers or fruit for centerpieces

Preparation:

1. Spread newspapers on the work area.
2. Pour tempera paint into several shallow trays.

Directions:

Have students dip the sponges in the paint, and then press them gently around the edges of their Place Mat activity sheets to make a border.

While the paint dries, let students create pretty centerpieces with flowers or fruit. Then have students arrange their place mats around the table. Read the poem aloud. Ask students to say the poem and practice setting the table. Encourage them to learn good table manners and to make mealtimes happy times.

Decorate your place mat.
And make it a pretty sight.
Fork and napkin on the left,
Plate in the middle,
Knife, spoon, and glass on the right.

1–11 NUTRITION REVIEW SHEETS

This is a good time to review what the children have learned about nutrition.

Materials:

copies of the review sheets 1–11A through 1–11E
pencils

Directions:

Have copies of these review sheets available for the children. They may be used for review, as independent activities, or they may be placed in learning centers.

Activity Sheets for Section 1: Nutrition

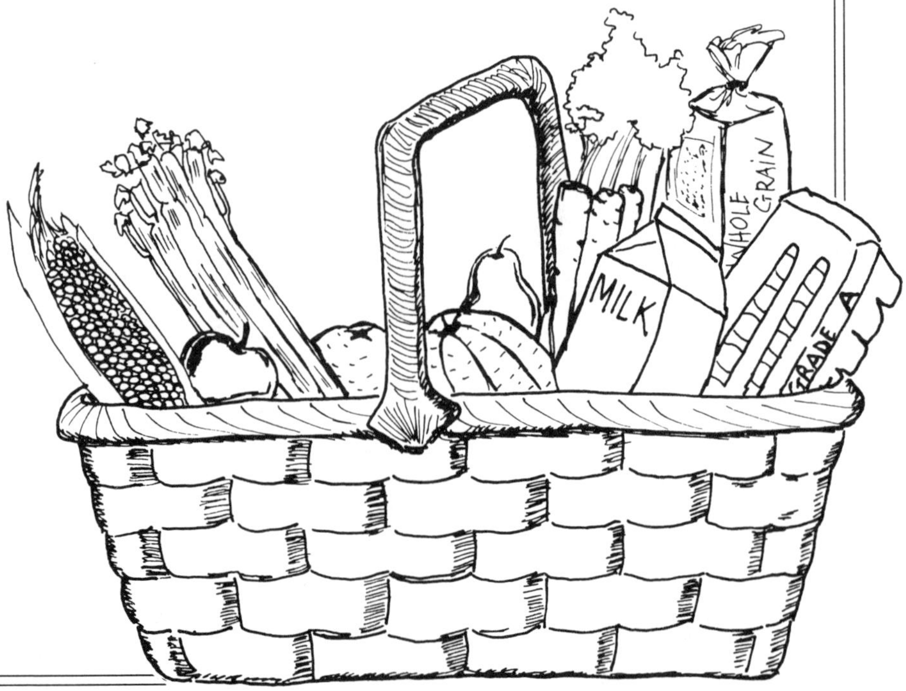

Name ______________________ Date ______________

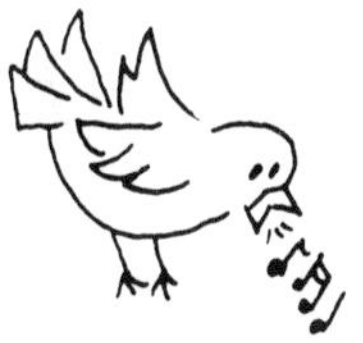

MILK GROUP

1–1A

Eat 3 servings a day.

Milk group foods help your teeth and bones grow strong.
Color the pictures.

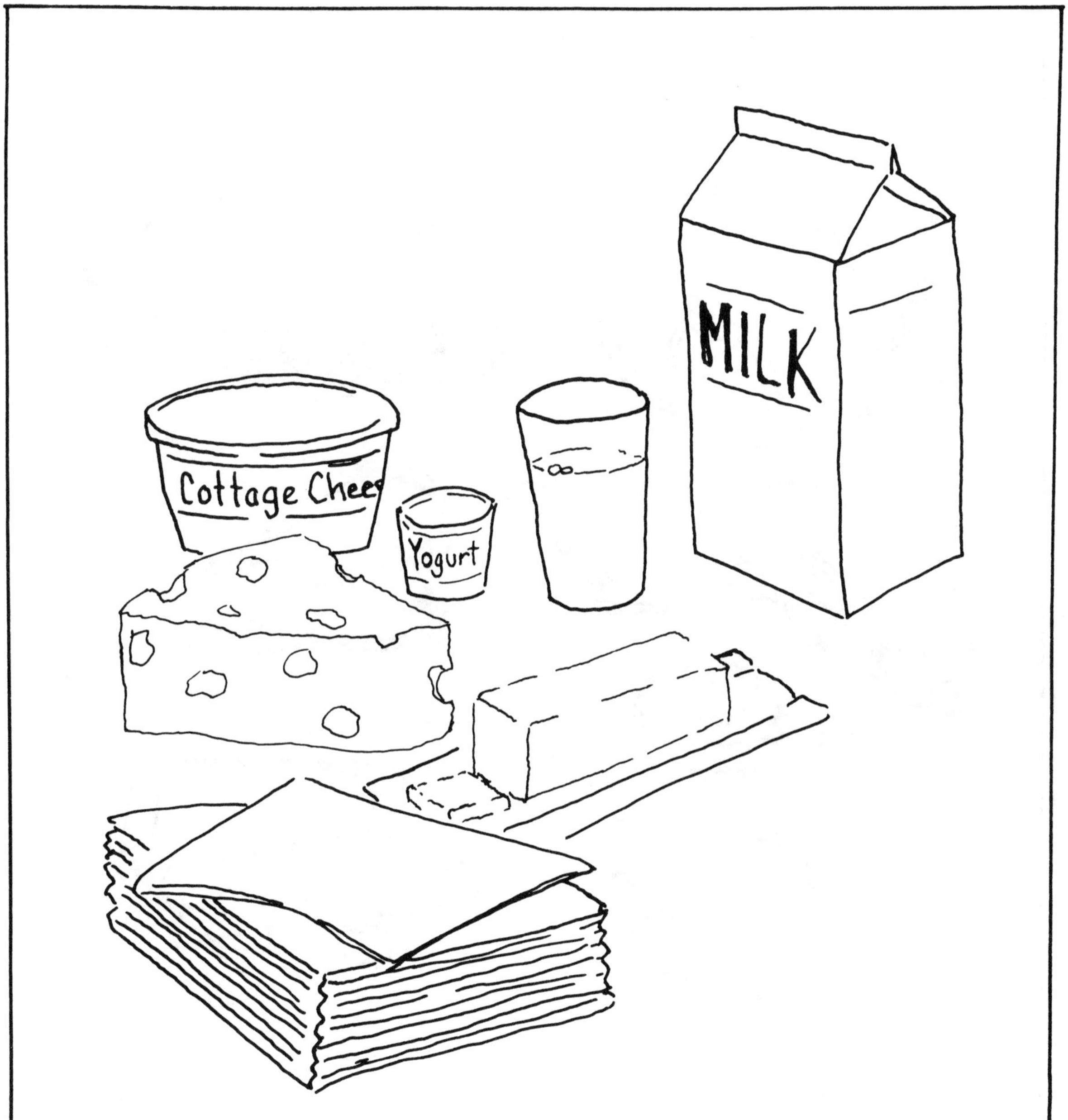

Name ______________________ Date ______________

FOOD PICTURES *1–2B*

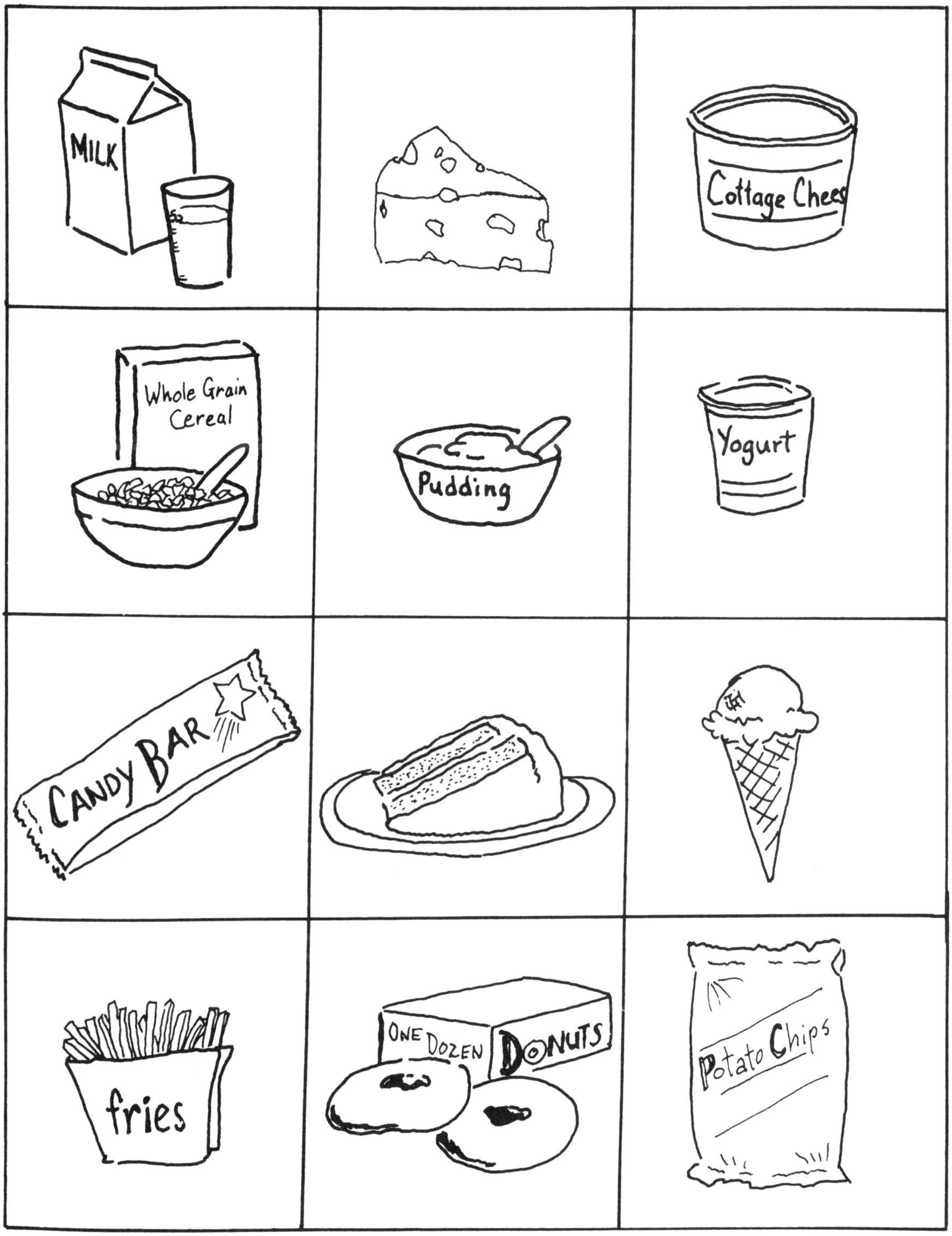

Name ______________________________ Date ________________

FOOD LOTTO GAME CARD *1–2C*

Name ________________________ Date ________________

PEAR PATTERN *1–4A*

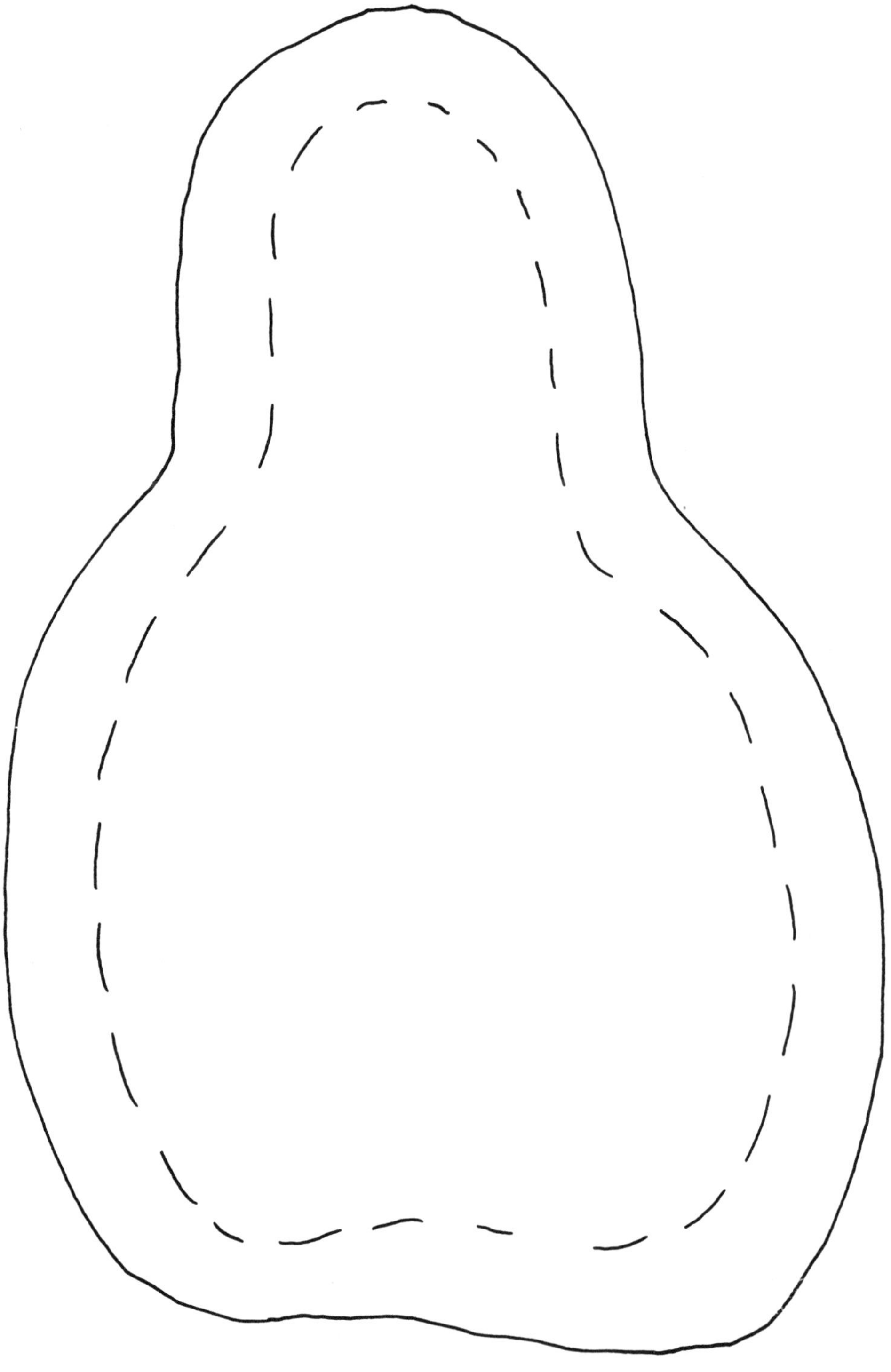

Name ______________________ Date ______________

APPLE PATTERN *1-4B*

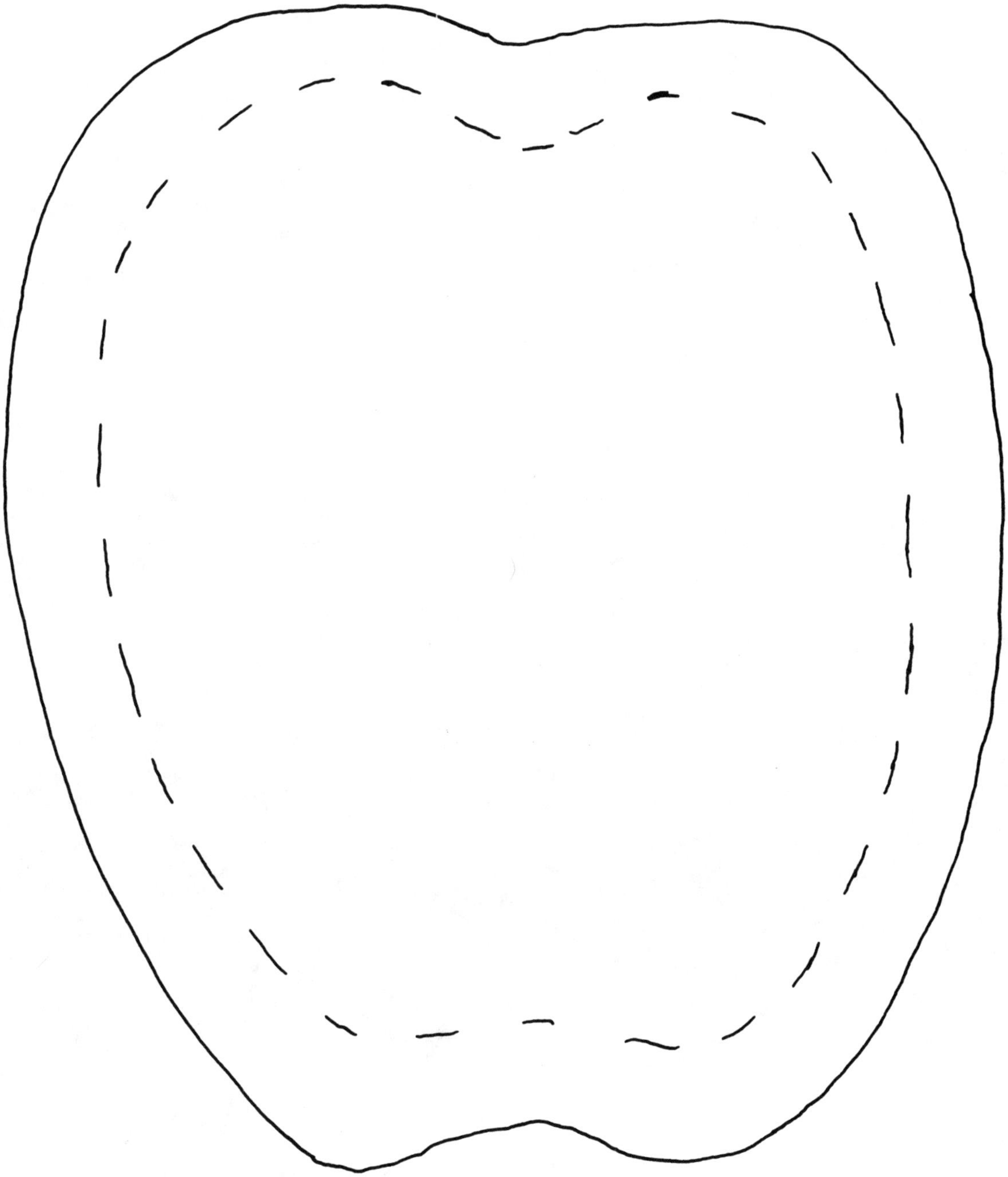

Name ________________________________ Date ____________________

CARROT PATTERN *1-4C*

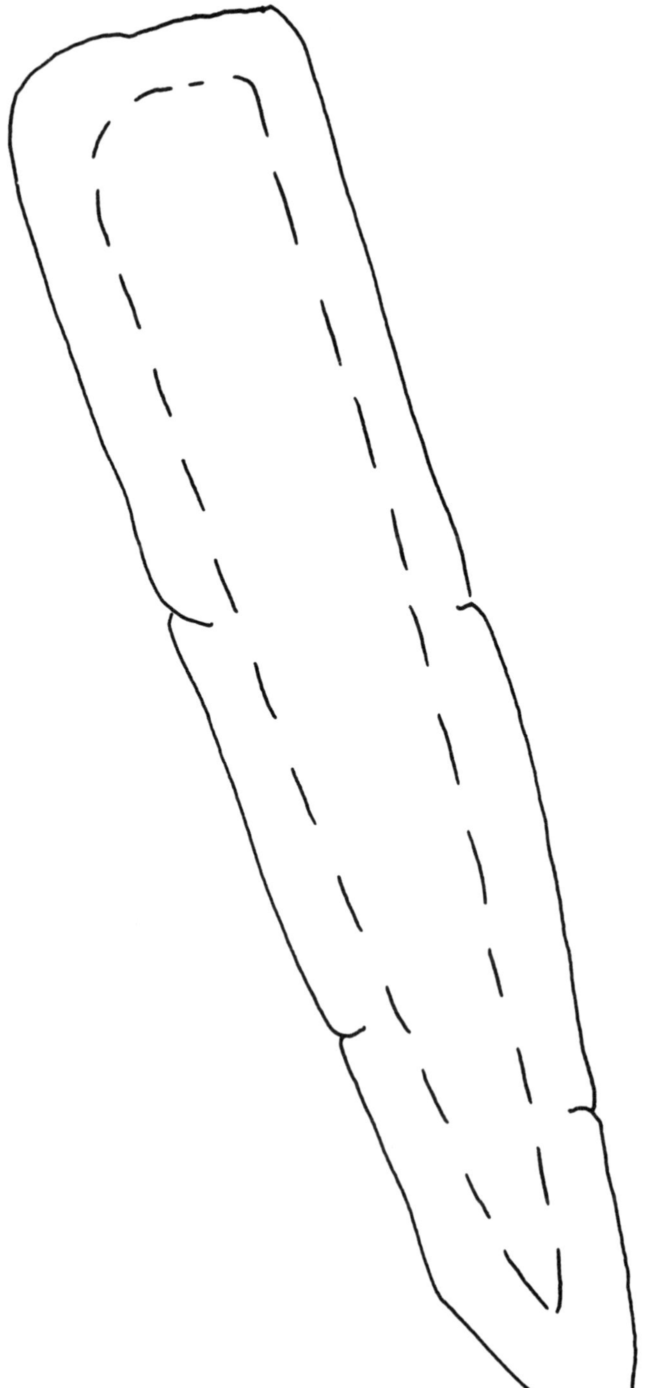

Name ______________________ Date ______________

ONION PATTERN *1-4D*

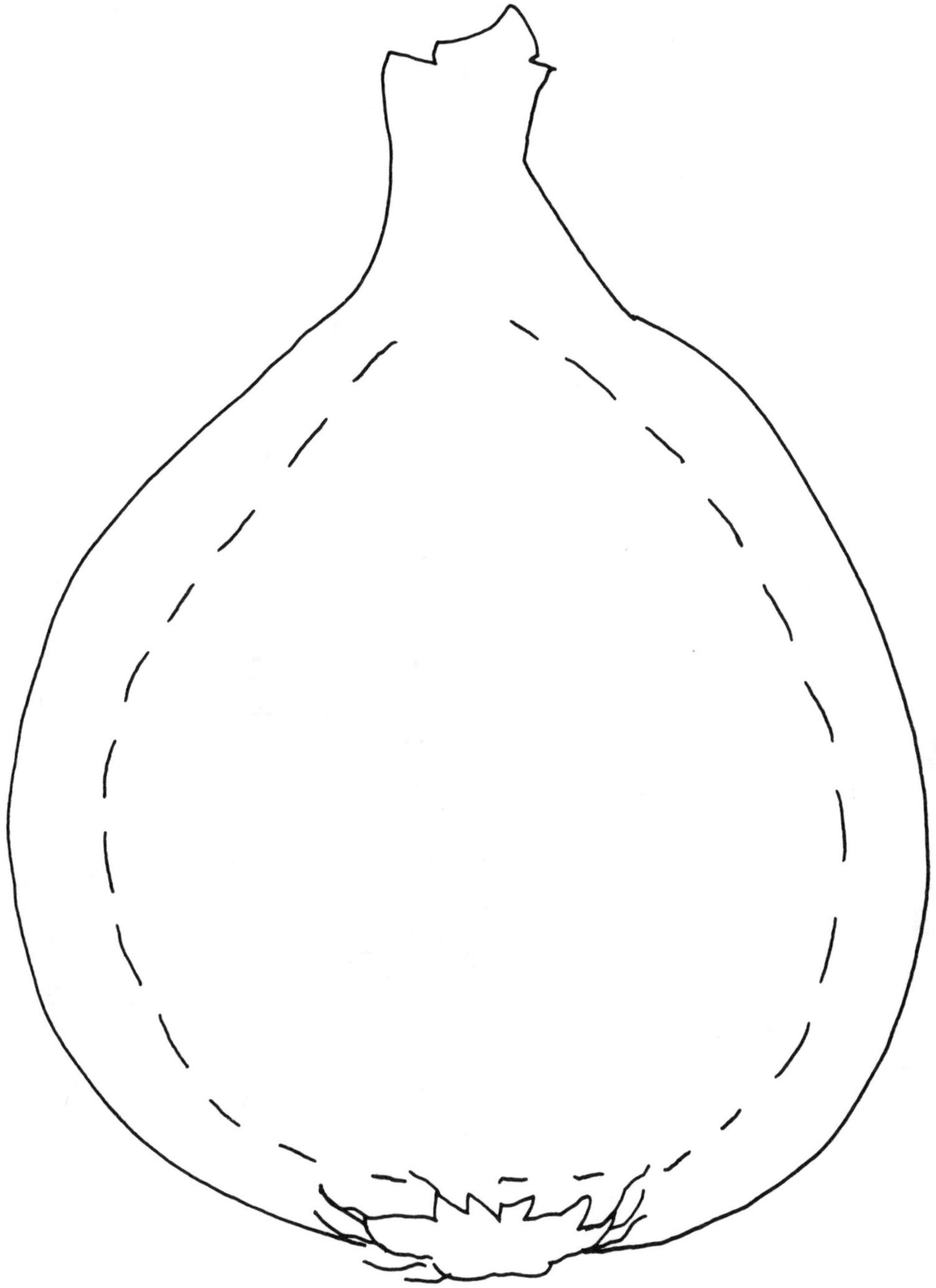

Name ______________________ Date ______________

VEGGIE VERSES

1–8A

1.	2.
3.	4.

Name ______________________________ **Date** ____________________

PLACE MAT *1–10A*

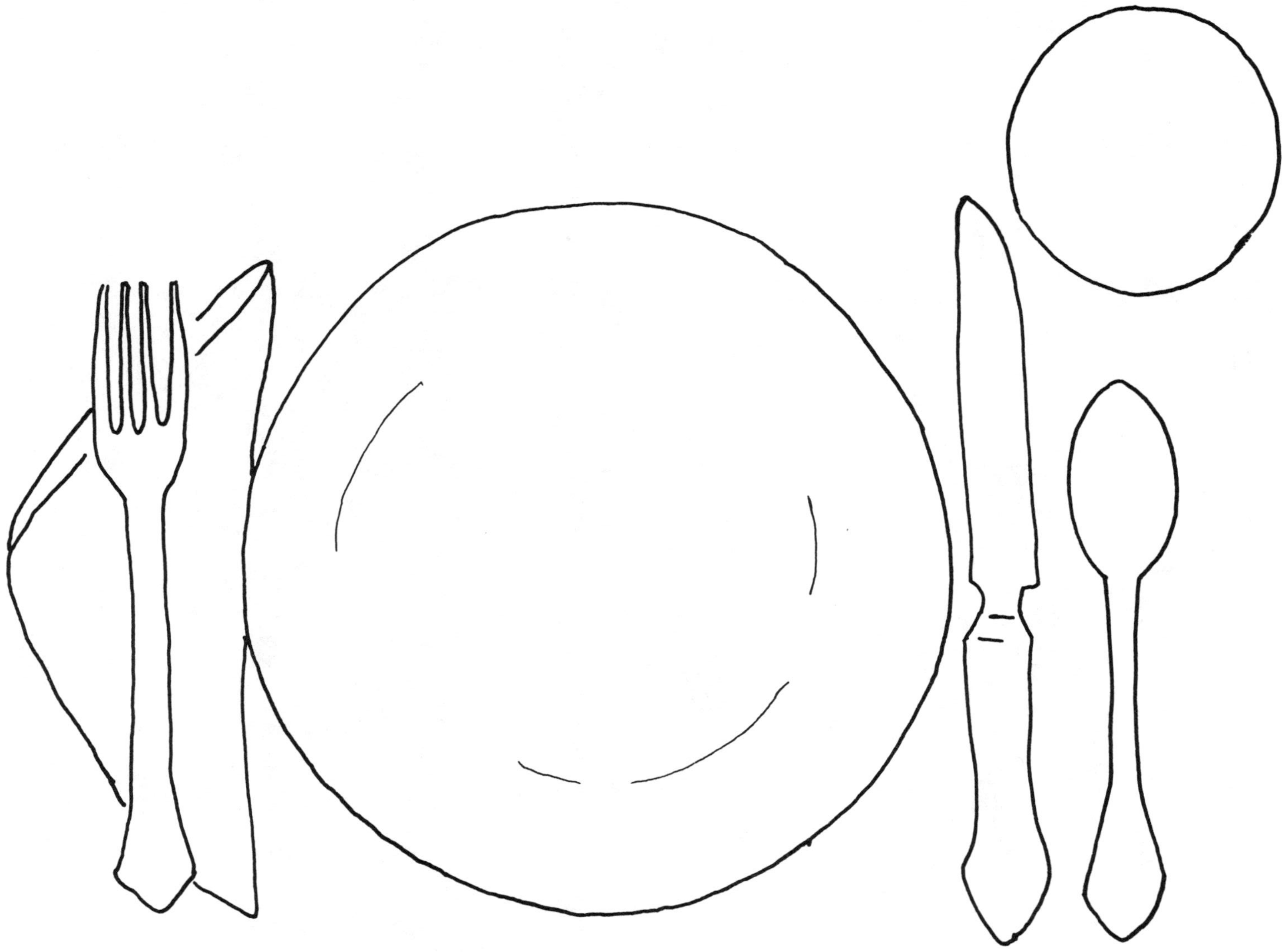

Name ______________________ Date ______________

FOLLOW THE FOOTPRINTS *1-11A*

Follow the footprints. Color the snacks that are good for you to eat. Cross out the ones that are not so good for you. At the end of the path, draw a healthy snack that you like to eat.

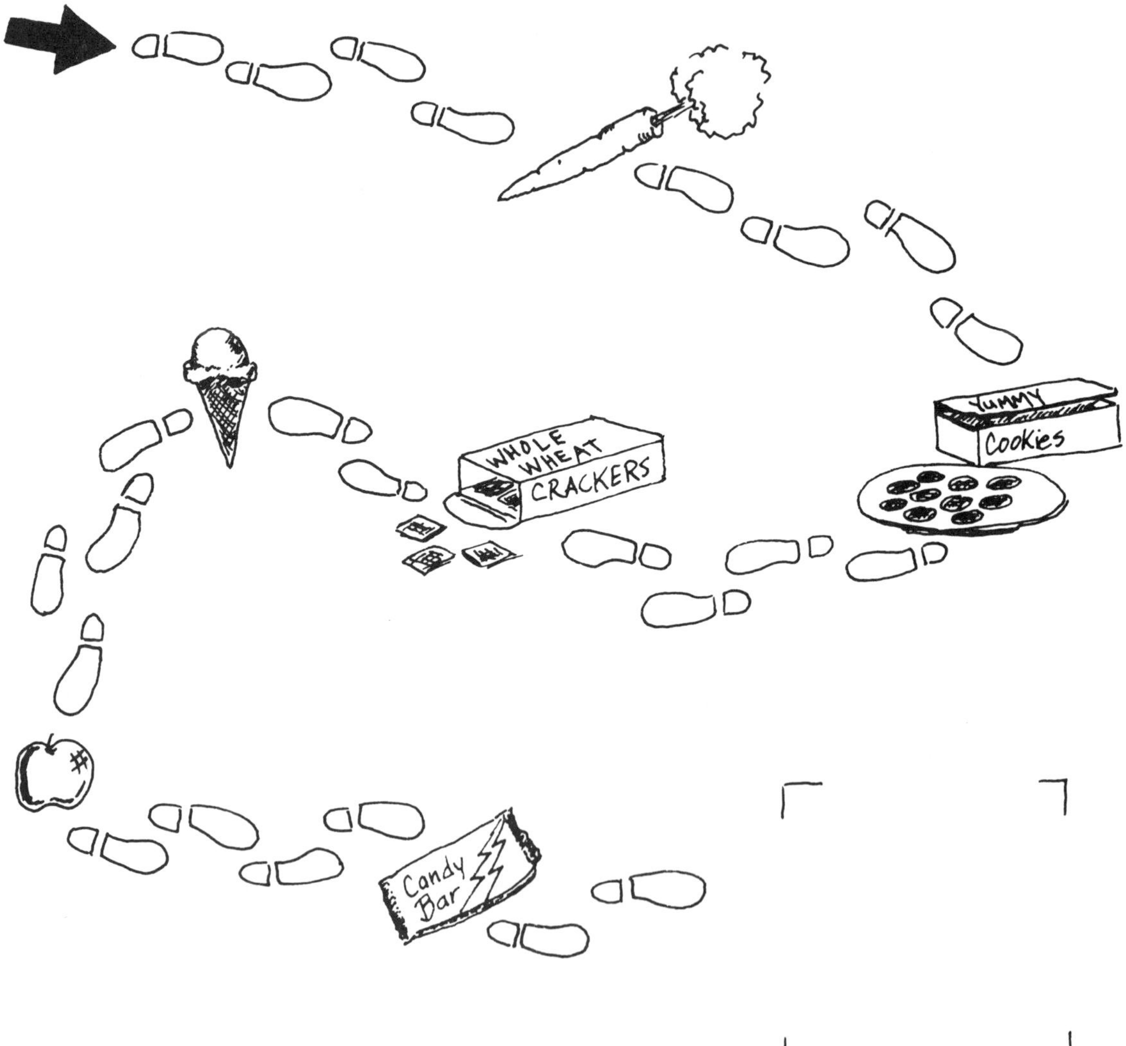

Name ______________________ Date ______________

PACK-A-LUNCH *1–11B*

Pretend to pack a healthy lunch. Draw the foods inside the lunch box. Be sure to draw one food from each of the four food groups.

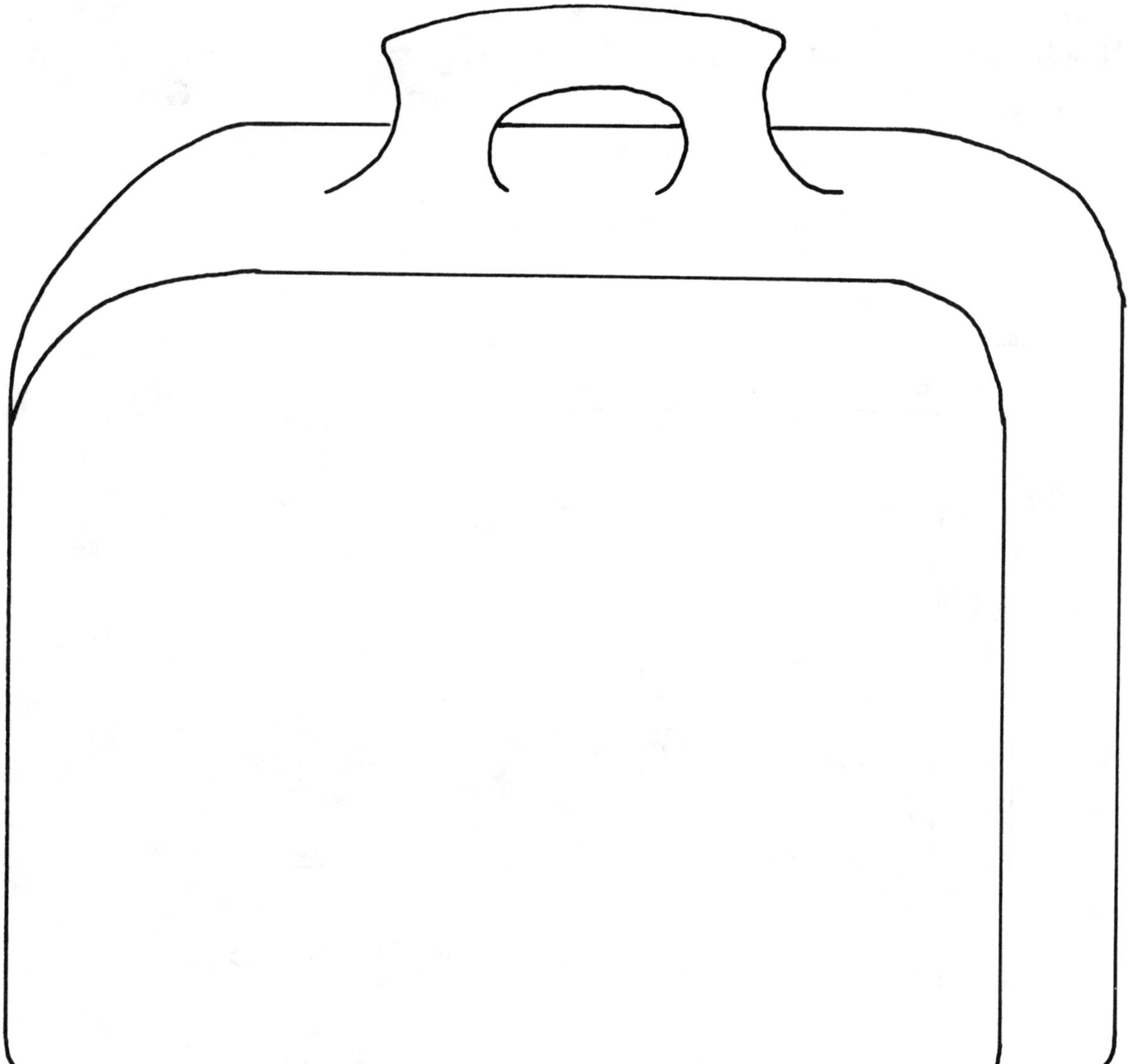

Name ______________________ Date ______________

FIND-A-FOOD *1–11C*

Look at the letters on the grocery bag. Find the hidden names of two foods from each food group. Circle the name of each food. Write the names of the foods.

Milk Group	Meat Group	Fruit-Vegetable Group	Bread-Cereal Group
__________	__________	__________	__________
__________	__________	__________	__________

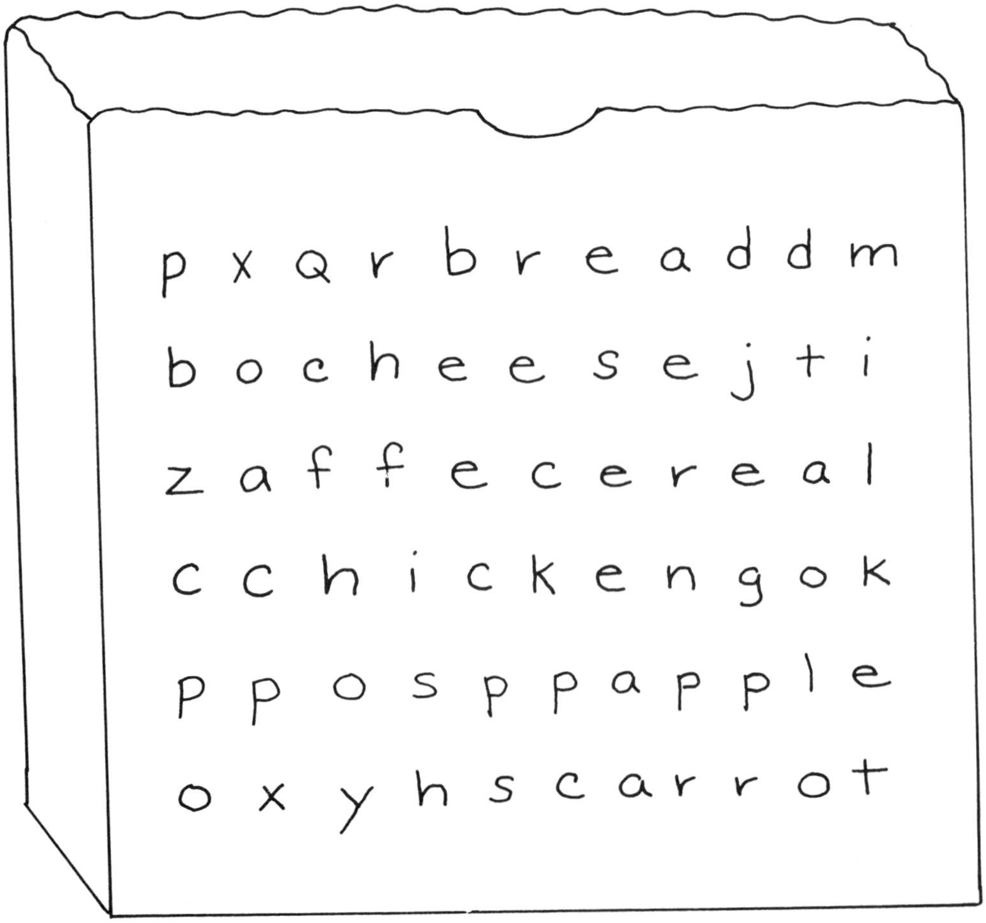

Name ______________________________ Date ______________

FAVORITE FOOD *1-11D*

Draw your favorite food on the plate. Write an "ad" telling about the food. Read your ad to the class.

______________ is my favorite food because ______________________________

____

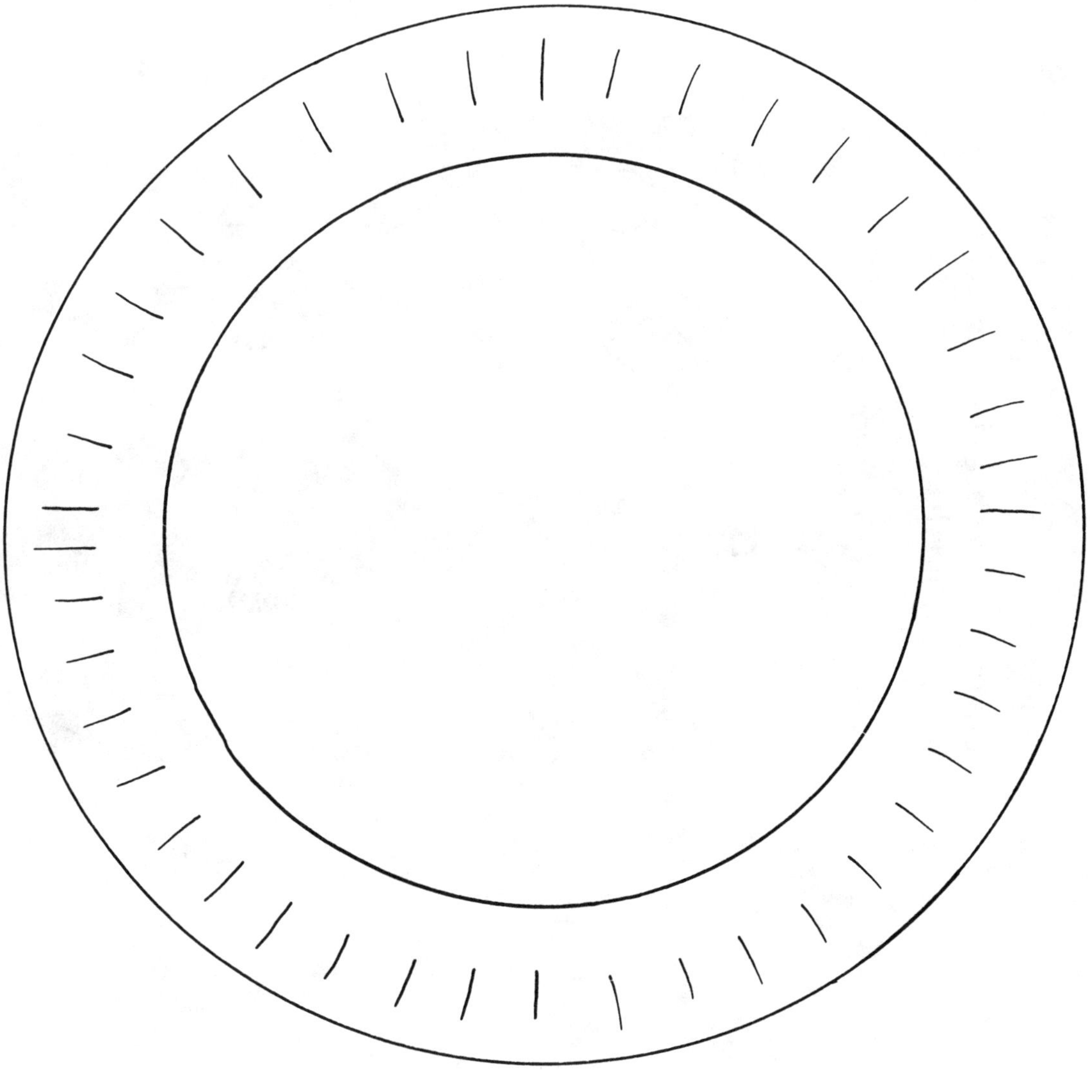

Name ______________________ Date ______________

GOOD BREAKFAST CODE *1–11E*

Eating a good breakfast gives you energy for the day. Use this code to find out some healthy foods to eat.

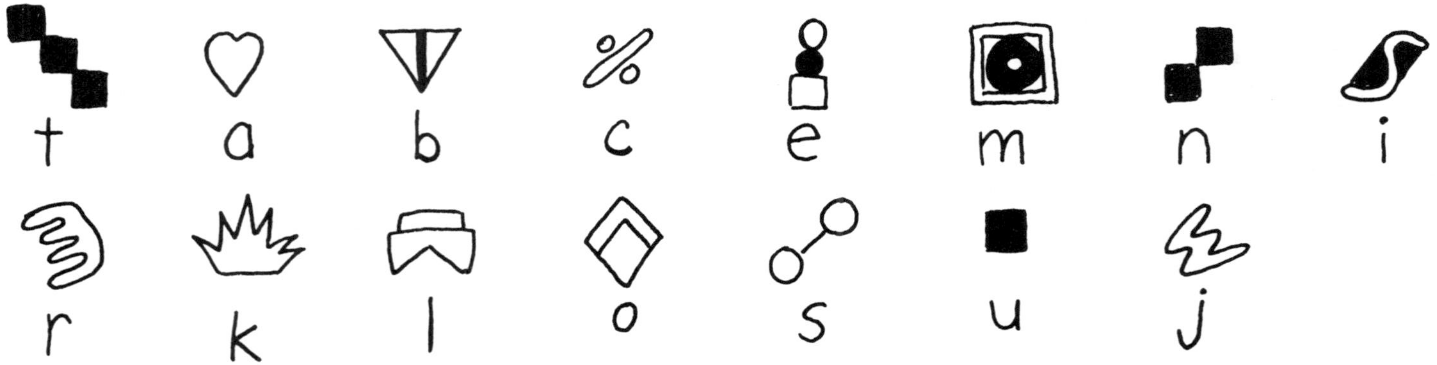

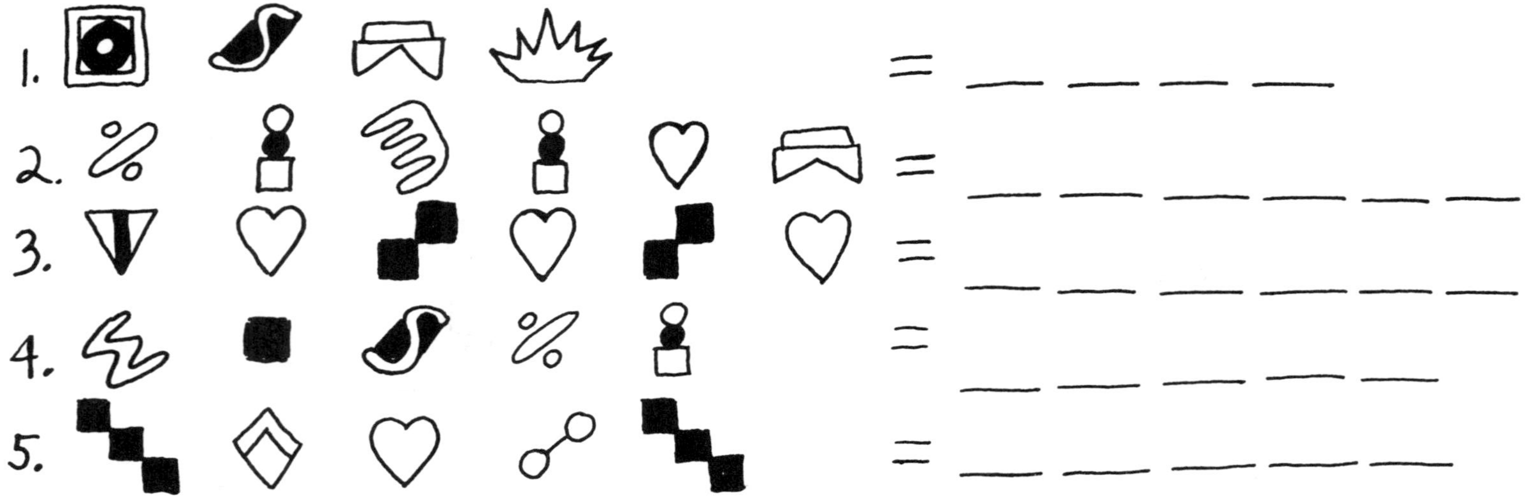

2 = RECIPES

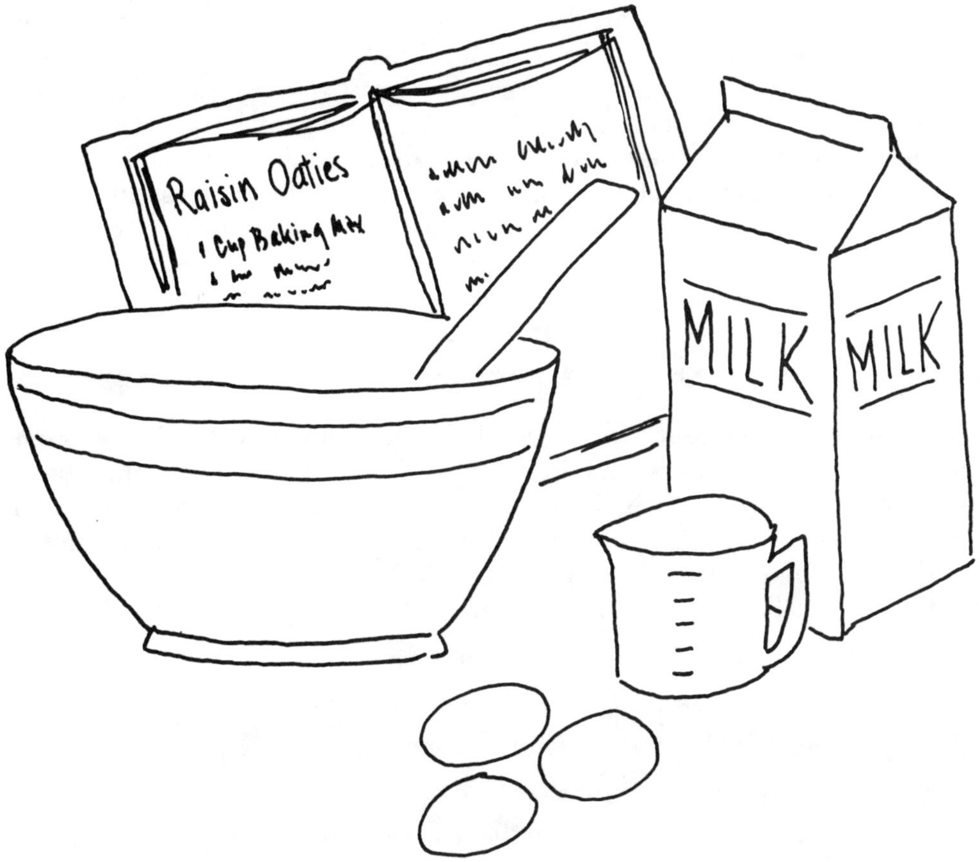

As your students take part in the preparation of nutritious foods, they will gain a sense of accomplishment and pride. Food preparation allows children to have fun and enjoy socializing with one another as they chop, measure, mix, cook, and eat. Children are more likely to enthusiastically taste and accept foods they have prepared themselves. Food preparation also gives students opportunities to build vocabulary, develop eye-hand coordination, practice fine motor skills, and improve reading, math, and communication skills.

The recipes that follow are designed to reinforce the concepts of good nutrition which were introduced in the Nutrition section. Because early nutritional habits have an important effect on later health, the recipes use low fat, low cholesterol, and low sodium ingredients whenever possible. Look for these products on the regular shelves or in the dietetic section of your supermarket, or in health food stores. The recipes are also low in sugar.

Stress hand-washing at the beginning of each food preparation experience. When recipes call for fresh vegetables or fruit, make sure the children scrub them thoroughly. Then demonstrate how to safely use utensils such as sharp knives, parers, or graters. Supervise the children carefully while they use utensils or appliances that could cause injury. Each recipe lists the utensils that will be needed as well as the ingredients. Keep the following supplies on hand in the classroom: paper plates and napkins; paper towels; plastic knives, forks, and spoons; measuring cups and spoons. In addition, some of the recipes call for a toaster oven, an oven, a blender, or an electric skillet. A picture symbol following each recipe shows the appliance that will be needed.

Be sure to involve all students in the food preparation process. Allow some students to measure ingredients while others add ingredients, and still others mix, beat, or stir the mixture. Four picture recipes are included which show students how to prepare individual portions. You may wish to enlarge and display each picture recipe, and discuss the numbered steps before students begin preparing the foods.

The activities in the Recipe section will help students:

- prepare nutritious foods for meals and snacks;
- sample a variety of foods that may be new to them:
- reinforce previously learned nutritional concepts;
- learn food preparation techniques;
- practice safe use of kitchen equipment and appliances.

Appliance Symbols:

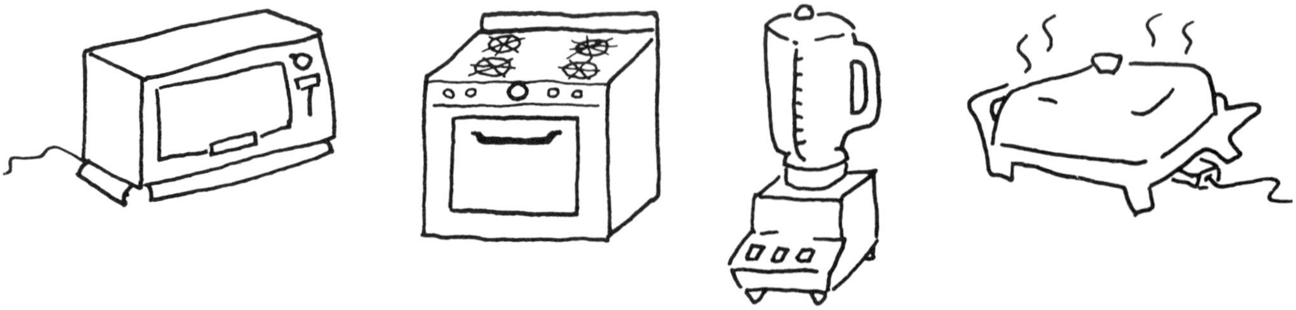

2–1 EDIBLE ART

Here's how to create a masterpiece that's good enough to eat!

You'll Need:

small plastic knives

whole grain bread (one slice per serving)

soft lowfat cream cheese or smooth unsalted peanut butter

some of these toppings:

raisins	shredded carrots
seedless grapes	banana slices
bean sprouts	pineapple chunks
pitted cherries	celery or carrot slices

Spread a layer of cream cheese or peanut butter on a slice of bread. Gently press on some of the toppings to create a design or a face. Compare creations, and then enjoy them as a nutritious snack.

2–2 RAISIN OATIES

These cookies are tasty as well as nutritious.

You'll Need:

- 1 cup baking mix
- 1½ cups quick-cooking oats
- ½ cup oat bran
- ½ tsp. cinnamon
- 1 cup brown sugar
- 2 egg whites
- ⅓ cup vegetable oil
- ½ cup nonfat milk
- 1 tsp. vanilla
- 1 cup raisins

- large mixing bowl
- small mixing bowl
- wooden mixing spoon
- measuring spoons
- measuring cups
- cookie sheets
- non-stick cooking spray
- potholders

Put baking mix, cinnamon, oatmeal, and oat bran in a large bowl. Mix well. Put egg whites in a small bowl and beat slightly. Stir in brown sugar, oil, milk, vanilla, and raisins. Blend well and stir into flour mixture. Spray the cookie sheets with non-stick cooking spray. Drop batter a teaspoon at a time onto cookie sheets. Bake at 375 degrees for 12 minutes. Cool for a few minutes. Makes 40 cookies.

Appliance Needed:

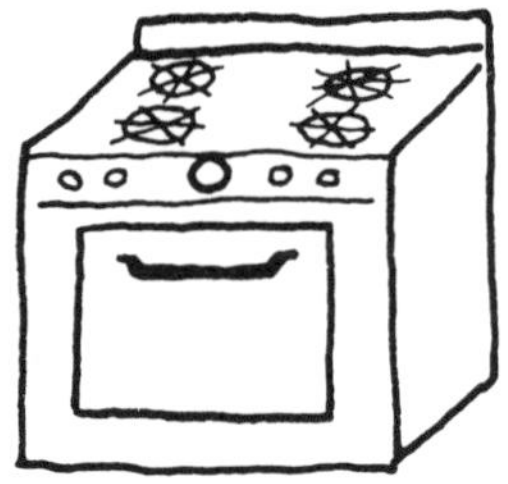

2–3 OATCAKES

Try this delicious and nutritious way to start the day.

You'll Need:

1 cup flour
1 cup quick-cooking oats
2 Tbsp. sugar
2 tsp. baking powder
1 tsp. baking soda
½ tsp. salt
1½ cups buttermilk
½ cup nonfat milk
2 Tbsp. vegetable oil
2 eggs
"lite" syrup

mixing bowl
rotary beater
measuring cups
measuring spoons
non-stick cooking spray
spatula

Put all ingredients except syrup in mixing bowl and beat with the rotary beater until smooth. Heat electric skillet. Spray skillet with non-stick cooking spray. Pour about ⅛ cup batter onto skillet for each pancake. When top bubbles, turn and cook the other side. Serve with "lite" syrup. Makes 20–24 oatcakes.

Appliance Needed:

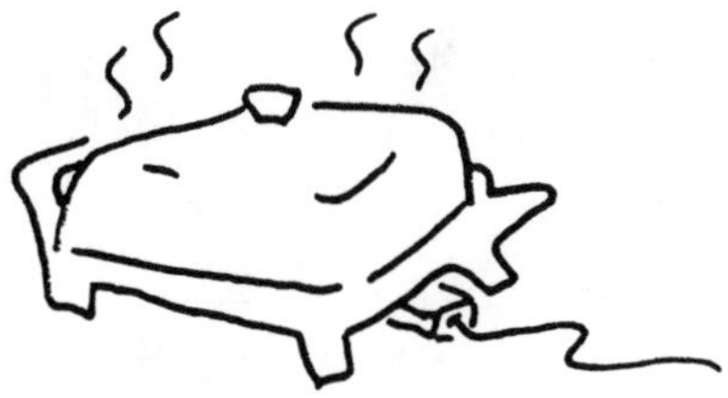

2–4 PRETTY PEACHES

Sweet, juicy peaches supply Vitamin C, fiber, and quick energy.

You'll Need:

29-ounce can of peach halves	baking sheet
lemon juice	measuring cup
¼ cup sugar	measuring spoon
2 tsp. ground cinnamon	spatula
	can opener

Drain peach halves and arrange on baking sheet, cut side up. Sprinkle with lemon juice. Mix sugar and cinnamon together and sprinkle on peaches. Broil until golden brown. Makes 8–10 servings.

Appliance Needed:

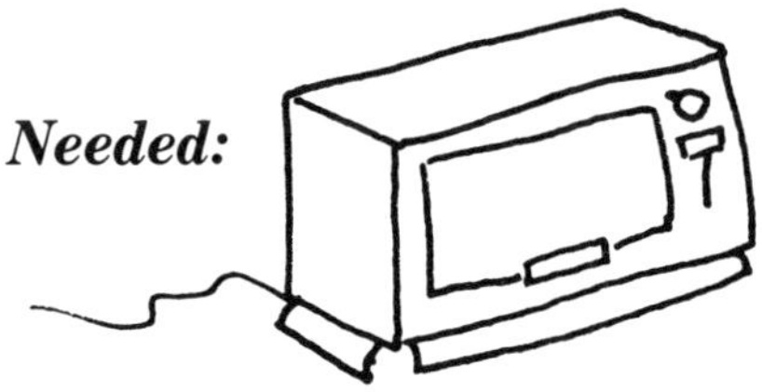

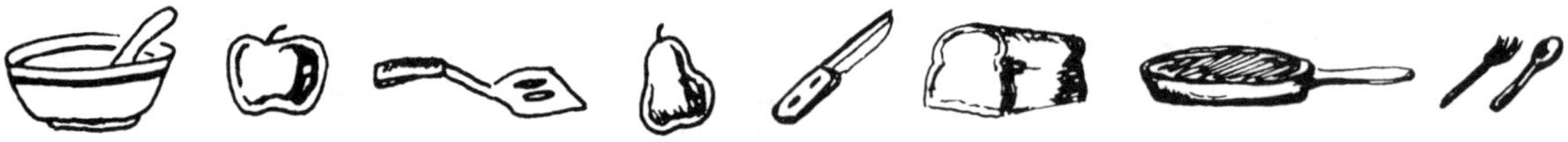

2–5 MUNCH, CRUNCH LUNCH

Children enjoy foods that make noise. Help students prepare this noisy meal.

You'll Need:

- apples, cabbage, carrots, celery, cucumbers, jicama, raw potatoes
- crisp pickles
- whole wheat crackers
- unsweetened crunchy cereals
- sharp knife
- two large plates
- paper towels
- chopping board

Wash and dry the fruits and vegetables. Carefully cut them into small slices. Cut the pickles into small slices. Arrange foods on a large plate. Arrange a selection of cereals and crackers on another plate.

Have students put a piece of each food on their plates. Read the poem aloud as students taste each food separately. Ask them to describe the sound each food makes. Then have them name other noisy foods.

Take a bite.
Chew carefully.
Munch, munch, munch.
Take a bite
And hear the sound.
Crunch, crunch, crunch.
Take a bite.
It's neat to eat
A munch, crunch, lunch.

2–6 BANANA BERRY-GO-ROUND

This easy-to-make blender beverage is a nutritious breakfast. Eating a good breakfast gives children a lot of energy after a night of sleep and helps them concentrate in school.

You'll Need:

- 1 tsp. vanilla
- 1 cup nonfat milk
- ½ cup plain yogurt
- ¼ cup toasted wheat germ
- 4 large strawberries, fresh or frozen, unsweetened
- ¼ cup sugarless strawberry jam
- 1 medium banana

- measuring cup
- measuring spoons
- small plastic knives

Pour milk into blender. Add yogurt, wheat germ, vanilla, strawberries, and jam. Slice banana into the mixture. Cover and blend for 1½ minutes. Makes 24 ounces.

Appliance Needed:

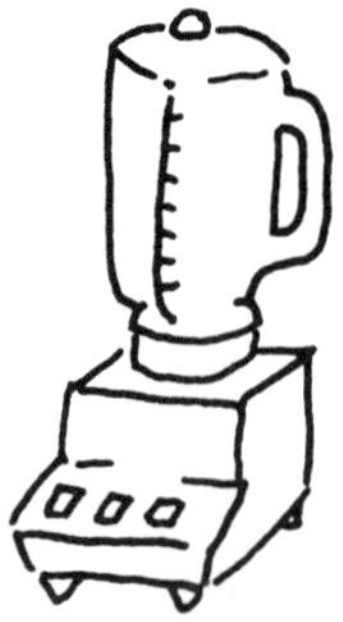

After enjoying the "Banana Berry-Go-Rounds," read this poem aloud and have students repeat it with you. Encourage students to eat a good breakfast every day.

Everybody needs to eat breakfast
To start the day off right.
A nutritious, delicious breakfast
Will keep me feeling bright.

2–7 PINEAPPLE PUDDING

This combination of pudding and pineapple makes a delicious dessert. Challenge students to think of other fruits that could be used in the pudding instead of pineapple.

You'll Need:

- sugar-free instant vanilla pudding mix (6-serving size)
- 8-ounce can of crushed pineapple in unsweetened juice
- 3 cups nonfat milk
- cinnamon
- large mixing bowl
- measuring cups
- rotary beater
- can opener

Pour nonfat milk into mixing bowl. Add pudding mix. Open can of pineapple but do not drain. Pour into bowl. Beat several minutes, until mixture thickens. Let set for 10 minutes. Spoon into bowls and sprinkle cinnamon on top of each serving. Makes ten ½ cup servings.

2–8 RAISINY-CARROT SALAD

Carrots are a good source of Vitamin A which is important to good health. It improves eyesight, keeps skin smooth and healthy, strengthens nails, and helps fight off infections and colds.

You'll Need:

- 8-ounce can crushed pineapple in unsweetened juice
- 4 medium carrots
- ½ cup raisins
- ¼ cup plain yogurt
- ¼ cup cholesterol-free mayonnaise
- ¼ cup toasted sunflower seeds

- large bowl
- parer
- grater
- measuring cups
- wooden spoon
- can opener

Wash and pare the carrots. Shred the carrots into the bowl. Stir in raisins. Drain pineapple and add to carrots. Stir in yogurt and mayonnaise. Sprinkle in sunflower seeds. Makes 2½ cups.

2–9 STIR-FRY CHICKEN

Stir up a quick and easy meal that includes meat, vegetables, and rice.

You'll Need:

- 2 lbs. pre-cooked boneless chicken, cut in 1-inch cubes
- 2 Tbsp. margarine
- 2 Tbsp. cornstarch
- 3½ cups low-sodium chicken broth
- 2 large carrots
- 4 Tbsp. lemon juice
- 6-ounce package frozen pea pods
- 3 cups dry instant rice

- wooden spoon
- measuring cups
- measuring spoons
- parer
- sharp knife
- chopping board

Wash and pare carrots, then cut in thin slices. Melt margarine in skillet. Saute chicken until lightly browned, about 5 minutes. Stir in cornstarch and cook 1 minute. Add broth, carrot slices, and lemon juice. Bring to a full boil, then simmer 1 to 2 minutes. Stir in pea pods and rice. Cover. Turn skillet off and let stand for 5 minutes. Stir mixture again before serving. Makes twelve ¾ cup servings.

Appliance Needed:

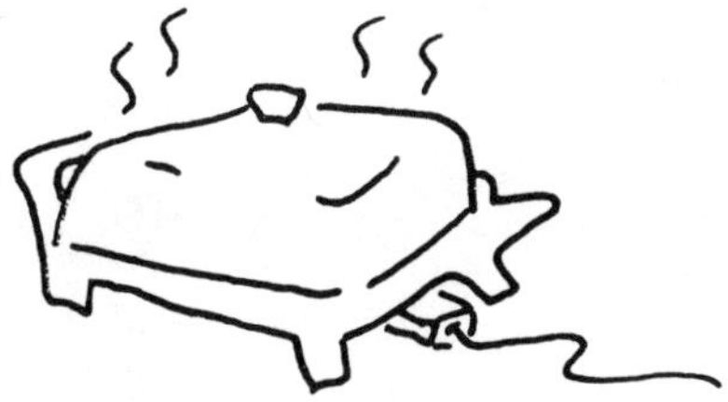

2–10 APPLE SANDWICHES

Apples are crisp, crunchy, and high in fiber. Prepare these unusual "apple sandwiches" with students.

APPLE-CHEESE SANDWICHES

You'll Need:

apples	apple corer
orange juice	shallow bowl
lowfat cheese slices	sharp knife
	chopping board

Wash apples thoroughly. Core the apples and slice, crosswise, to make apple rings. Pour orange juice into shallow bowl, and then dip the apple slices in the juice to keep them from turning brown. Place a slice of cheese between two apple rings to make a sandwich.

APPLE-RAISIN-PEANUT BUTTER SANDWICHES

You'll Need:

apples	apple corer
orange juice	shallow bowl
peanut butter	sharp knife
raisins	small plastic knives
	chopping board

Wash apples thoroughly. Core the apples and slice, crosswise, to make apple rings. Pour orange juice into shallow bowl, and then dip the apple slices in the juice to keep them from turning brown. Spread one apple ring with peanut butter and sprinkle on raisins. Top with another apple ring to make a sandwich.

2–11 APPLESAUCE

You can use Gravenstein, McIntosh, Delicious, or other varieties of apples to prepare this tasty treat.

You'll Need:

1 apple per serving	sharp knife
1 Tbsp. water per serving	measuring spoons
1 tsp. sugar per serving	mixing spoon
1 tsp. cinnamon	potato masher
dash of salt (optional)	chopping board

Wash apples thoroughly. Peel and core apples and cut them into small pieces. Put apples, water, and sugar in an electric skillet. Stir in cinnamon and salt. Simmer until apples are tender, stirring occasionally. Add more water if necessary. For smoother applesauce, mash the apple mixture with a potato masher until it is the desired consistency.

Appliance Needed:

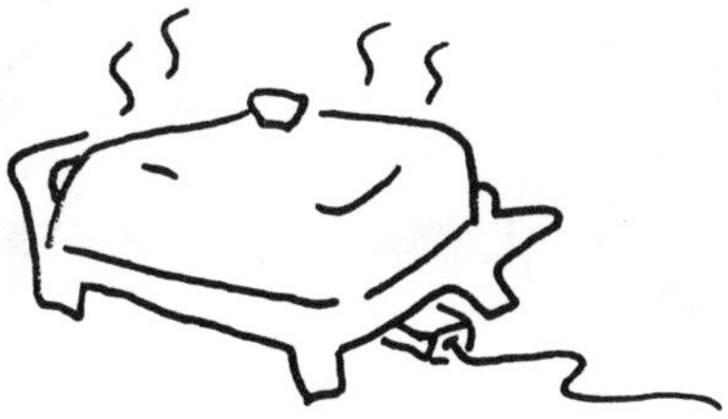

2–12 FROZEN YOGURT YUMMIES

Yogurt yummies provide an excellent source of protein for growing bodies.

You'll Need:

- 8-ounce carton of plain yogurt
- 6-ounce can frozen juice concentrate, thawed
- spoon
- 6 small paper cups (3-ounce size)
- 6 craft sticks
- freezer

Pour thawed juice into blender. Add yogurt. Blend until smooth. Pour into cups until ⅛-inch from top. Put in freezer. Add a craft stick to each cup when mixture starts to freeze. Peel off paper before eating. Makes 6 yogurt yummies.

Appliance Needed:

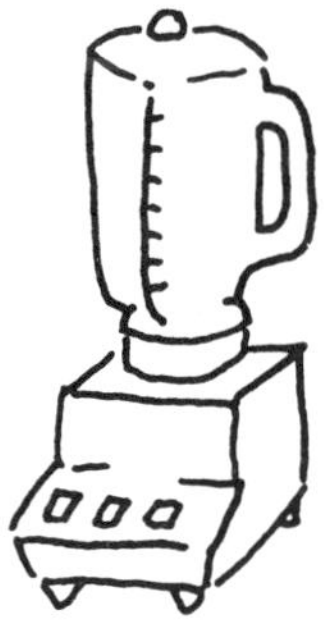

2–13 TUNA TRIANGLES

Try a tasty tuna triangle today. The students will love preparing these nutritious seafood snacks. Encourage them to eat several servings of fish every week. It is a good source of protein which helps bodies grow strong.

You'll Need:

- 6½-ounce can of water-packed tuna
- ½ cup nonfat yogurt
- 1 Tbsp. cholesterol-free mayonnaise
- ¼ cup unsalted sunflower seeds
- ¼ cup raisins
- 1 Tbsp. lemon juice
- 1 small carrot
- salt-free seasoning
- alfalfa sprouts (optional)
- whole grain bread

- can opener
- mixing bowl
- mixing spoon
- measuring spoons
- measuring cups
- sharp knife
- parer
- grater
- small plastic knives

Drain tuna and put in mixing bowl. Stir in yogurt, mayonnaise, sunflower seeds, and raisins. Add lemon juice to tuna mixture. Wash and pare carrot. Grate and add to tuna. Season and mix well. Cut each bread slice into 4 small triangles and spread tuna mixture on each one. Sprinkle with sprouts, if desired. Makes 1½ cups tuna mixture.

2–14 FRUIT BITES

These easy-to-make fruit bites are fun to prepare and delicious to eat.

You'll Need:

- 1 cup dates, pitted
- 1 cup prunes, pitted
- 1 cup dried apricots
- ½ cup nuts, finely chopped

- measuring cup
- ruler
- scissors
- sharp knife
- mixing bowl
- mixing spoon
- aluminum foil
- covered container
- chopping board

Cut aluminum foil into forty-eight 3½″ squares. Chop all the fruit into small pieces and put into bowl. Add nuts and mix well. Roll mixture into 1″ fruit balls. Put each ball on a piece of foil. Lay one edge of foil over the ball, then roll the ball to the other edge. Twist the open ends of foil in opposite directions. Put fruit bites in a covered container and store in the refrigerator. Makes about 48 pieces.

2–15 NEW FOOD NEWS SALAD

Encourage students to try new foods occasionally. Read the poem aloud, then help the students prepare this salad with some different vegetables.

Try a new food just for fun
Soon it may be your favorite one.

You'll Need:

- 1 cup raw broccoli
- 1 medium raw zucchini
- 1 cup raw cauliflower
- 1 small jar artichoke hearts
- 1 Tbsp. parsley flakes
- 1 tsp. lemon juice
- salt-free seasoning
- 3 Tbsp. light French dressing
- paper towels
- large bowl
- wooden spoon
- measuring cups
- measuring spoons
- sharp knife
- chopping board

Wash broccoli, zucchini, and cauliflower. Remove leaves and dry thoroughly with paper towels. Cut broccoli and cauliflower into flowerets. Slice zucchini into sticks. Put into bowl. Drain artichoke hearts and cut into bite-size pieces. Sprinkle in parsley flakes, seasoning, and lemon juice. Stir in salad dressing and toss gently. Makes $2\frac{3}{4}$ cups.

2–16 DIPPERS

Raw vegetables make a terrific taste treat for munching. Help the students wash, cut, and chop vegetables for this nutritious high fiber meal. Have them chant this verse while they work.

Veggies, veggies
Crispy and crunchy.
Wash them, peel them
Dip them for lunchy.

You'll Need:

An assortment of the following vegetables:

- beets
- broccoli
- carrots
- cauliflower
- cherry tomatoes
- cucumbers
- jicama
- green beans
- green pepper
- yams

- sharp knife
- parer
- chopping board
- paper towels
- large platter

Wash and dry beets, carrots, jicama, and yams. Peel jicama and yams and cut into thin slices. Pare carrots and cut into slices. Wash and dry broccoli and cauliflower. Chop into chunks. Wash and dry tomatoes. Remove stems. Wash and dry green pepper. Cut in half, remove seeds and cut into thin strips. Wash and dry string beans and chop off ends. Wash and dry cucumbers and thinly slice. Arrange vegetables on platter.

2–17 DELIGHTFUL DIP

Help the students make this delicious dip for their crispy vegetable dippers.

You'll Need:

- 8-ounce carton of plain nonfat or lowfat yogurt
- 3 ounces Neufchâtel cream cheese, softened
- 1 tsp. lemon juice
- ½ tsp. salt-free seasoning
- ¼ cup cholesterol-free mayonnaise
- 1 Tbsp. parsley flakes
- ¼ cup light French dressing

- small mixing bowl
- measuring cups
- measuring spoons
- wooden spoon

Put yogurt, cream cheese, lemon juice, mayonnaise, and dressing into bowl. Blend well. Sprinkle in seasoning and parsley. Blend. Makes 1½ cups.

2–18 GOLDEN BROWN COTTAGE CHEESE CAKES

Morning, noon, or night these make a delicious meal.

You'll Need:

- 1 cup lowfat cottage cheese
- 8 Tbsp. light corn oil margarine
- 2 eggs
- ½ tsp. baking powder
- 1 cup flour
- ½ cup nonfat milk
- cinnamon
- small jar of applesauce

- large mixing bowl
- measuring cups
- measuring spoons
- wooden spoon
- tablespoon
- non-stick cooking spray
- spatula

Put cottage cheese and margarine into bowl. Blend until creamy. Stir in eggs. Add flour and baking powder and mix well. Gradually stir in the milk. Lightly spray skillet with non-stick spray, and heat to medium. Drop the batter by tablespoonfuls onto skillet. Cook until golden brown, turning over once. Sprinkle with cinnamon and top with applesauce. Makes about 24 small cakes.

Appliance Needed:

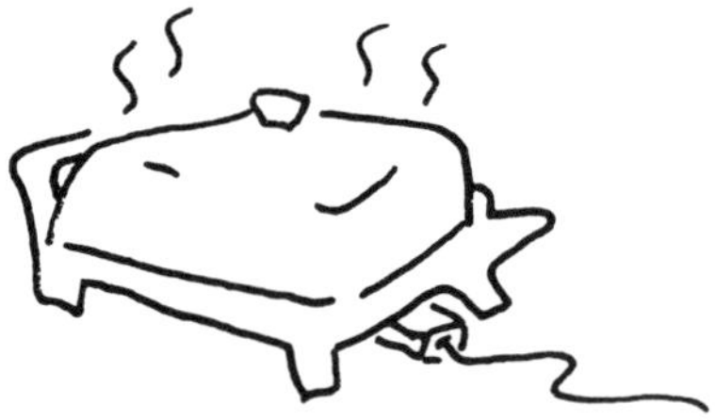

2–19 TASTY TATERS

Enjoy a terrific treat with tasty taters.

You'll Need:

large potato	sharp knife
vegetable oil	fork
salt-free seasoning	baking sheet
	paper towels
	non-stick cooking spray
	chopping board

Spray baking sheet with non-stick spray. Wash and dry potato. Cut it in half the long way, then cut into ¼″ slices. Arrange on the baking sheet. Pour some vegetable oil onto a paper towel. Gently dab oil onto one side of potatoes. Lightly sprinkle with salt-free seasoning. Bake in 350-degree oven for approximately 25 minutes. Makes about 24 slices.

Appliance Needed:

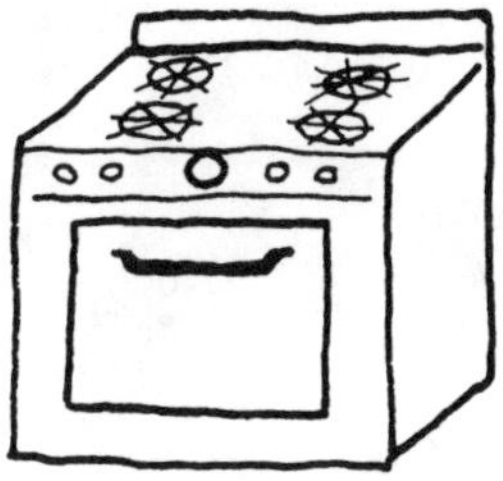

2–20 TASTY TOASTY PUMPKIN SEEDS

Nuts and seeds provide an excellent source of protein. Help students prepare this tasty toasty treat.

You'll Need:

- large pumpkin
- salt-free seasoning

- knife
- baking sheet
- strainer
- wooden spoon
- paper towels
- non-stick cooking spray

Cut open pumpkin, scoop seeds into strainer, and rinse with warm water. Dry seeds on paper towels. Lightly spray baking sheet with non-stick spray. Spread seeds on baking sheet and sprinkle with seasoning. Cook in 250-degree oven, stirring occasionally. Roast until lightly browned or about 45 minutes.

Appliance Needed:

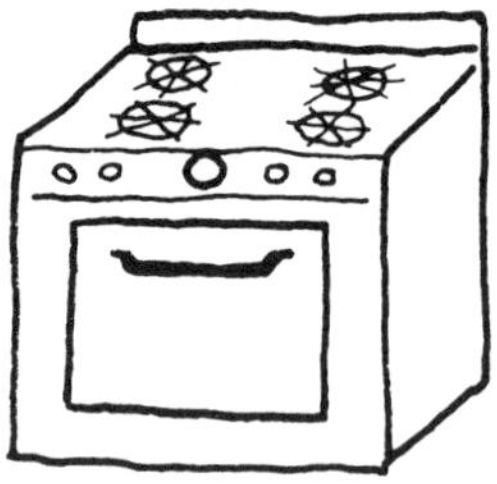

2–21 PITA PIECES

Pita pieces offer good nutritional value.

You'll Need:

package of whole wheat pitas
1 cup red cabbage
1 large celery stalk
2 medium carrots
1 medium tomato
small green pepper
1 small cucumber
¼ lb. thinly sliced turkey breast
light salad dressing
cholesterol-free mayonnaise

chopping board
sharp knife
parer
measuring cups
seven small bowls
seven spoons
paper towels

Cut pitas in half and warm in skillet. Wash and dry all vegetables. Cut cabbage, tomato, and cucumber into thin slices. Cut ends from celery and carrots. Chop celery into small pieces. Pare and cut carrots into thin rings. Cut green pepper in half, remove seeds, and cut into thin strips. Put turkey and vegetables into separate bowls. Put a slice of turkey in each pita half, and then add vegetables. Top with a little salad dressing or mayonnaise. Each half of a pita equals one serving.

Appliance Needed:

2–22 MAN-IN-THE-MOON-CAKES

This is a crunchy delicious way to add protein to a meal.

You'll Need:

- copies of Man-in-the-Moon Cake recipe (2–22A)
- ¼ cup part-skim mozzarella or other lowfat cheese per serving
- low-sodium rice cakes
- raisins
- grater
- baking sheet

Set out the ingredients and utensils in the order in which they will be used in the recipe. Help students follow the recipe directions. Have students add the Man-in-the-Moon Cake recipe to their "Here's to My Health" booklet file folders.

Appliance Needed:

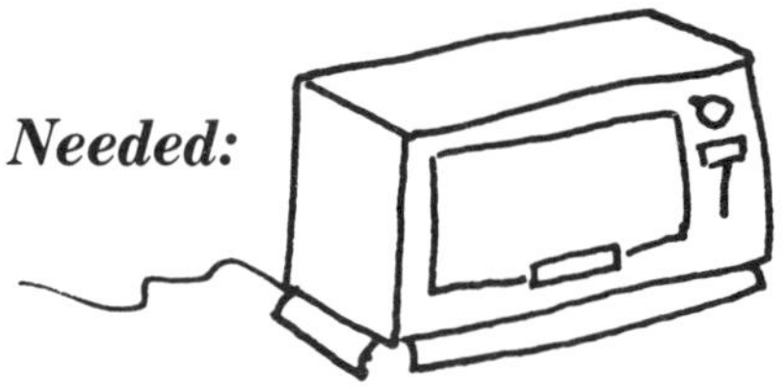

After students prepare their Man-in-the-Moon Cakes, read this poem aloud and have them repeat it with you. Then enjoy the Man-in-the-Moon Cakes together.

Man-in-the-Moon,
Tell me please.
Are you really
Made of cheese?

Man-in-the-Moon,
Yes, it's true.
I can make a
Meal of you.

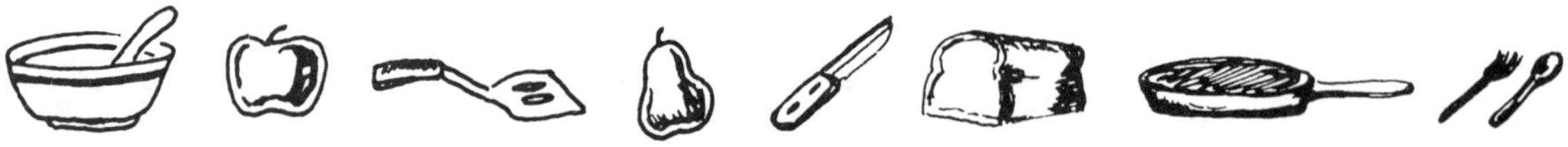

2–23 BACKPACK SNACKS

TASTY TAKE-ALONGS

You'll Need:

1 cup shredded wheat squares
1 cup plain Cheerios™
1½ cups apple-cinnamon Cheerios™
½ cup raisins
1 cup dried banana chips

measuring cups
large paper bag
plastic sandwich bags

Put all ingredients in paper bag. Close the bag and shake well. Put ¼ cup of mix into each sandwich bag. Makes sixteen ¼ cup servings.

STACKER CRACKERS

You'll Need:

copies of Stacker Cracker recipe (2–23A)
unsalted peanut butter
low-sodium crackers
bananas

small plastic knives
plastic sandwich bags

Set out the ingredients and utensils in the order in which they will be used in the recipe. Help students follow the recipe directions. Have them put their Stacker Crackers in plastic sandwich bags. Then have them add the Stacker Cracker recipe to their "Here's to My Health" booklet file folders.

2–24 HIKE UP A HILL

It takes a lot of energy to hike up a hill, so help students prepare healthy snacks to take along. After preparing "Backpack Snacks" (see recipe 2–23A), read the poem aloud and have students act it out. Then sit down together to enjoy a backpack picnic.

Put on your backpack.
Let's hike up a hill.
We'll hike and hike
And hike until
Someone gets tired
And it's time to rest.
Look at that bird.
Do you see its nest?
Let's lie on our backs
And stare at the sky
Looking for pictures
As clouds roll by.
Let's hike some more now
Through rocks and tall trees
Watching their branches
Sway in the breeze.
We'll climb up higher
And then we'll stop.
Hooray! We did it.
We hiked to the top.
It's time to relax
And look all around
With a backpack picnic
Spread on the ground.

2–25 TURKEY ROLLAROUNDS

Good-tasting sandwiches can be made without using bread. Help students prepare these "rollaround sandwiches."

You'll Need:

- copies of Turkey Rollaround recipe (2–25A)
- thin turkey slices
- thin Swiss or mozzarella cheese slices
- bunch of small carrots
- cholesterol-free mayonnaise
- head of lettuce or spinach
- parer
- sharp knife
- chopping board
- small plastic knives

Wash and dry lettuce. Break off lettuce leaves. Wash and pare carrots. Cut carrots lengthwise into 3″ pieces.

Set out the ingredients and utensils in the order in which they will be used in the recipe. Help students follow the recipe directions. Have students add the Turkey Rollaround recipe to their "Here's to My Health" booklet file folders.

After students eat their Turkey Rollarounds, ask them to name other foods they might use to make "rollaround sandwiches."

2–26 MINI-MUFFIN PIZZA

Try this favorite snack made the healthy, nutritious way.

You'll Need:

- copies of Mini-Muffin Pizza recipe (2–26A)
- English muffins
- low sodium tomato sauce or ketchup
- ¼ cup part-skim mozzarella or other lowfat cheese per serving
- mushrooms
- green pepper
- grater
- small plastic knives
- sharp knife
- chopping board
- can opener (for tomato sauce)

Wash mushrooms and green pepper. Slice mushrooms. Chop green pepper into small pieces. Split each English muffin into two halves.

Set out the ingredients and utensils in the order in which they will be used in the recipe. Help students follow the recipe directions. Have students add the Mini-Muffin Pizza recipe to their "Here's to My Health" booklet file folders.

Appliance Needed:

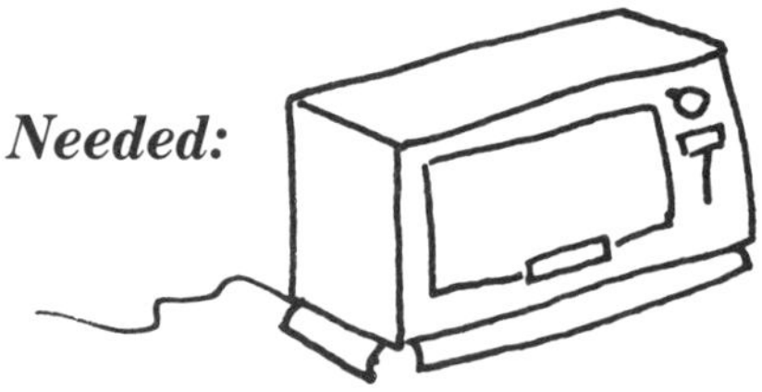

Activity Sheets for Section 2: Recipes

2–22A Man-in-the-Moon Cake
2–23A Stacker Crackers
2–25A Turkey Rollaround
2–26A Mini-Muffin Pizza

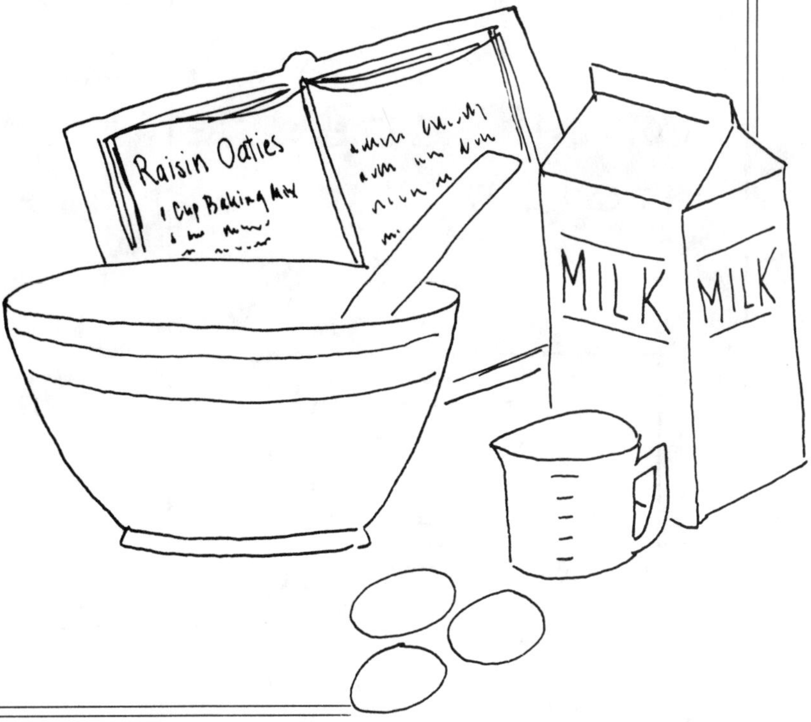

Name ______________________ Date ______________

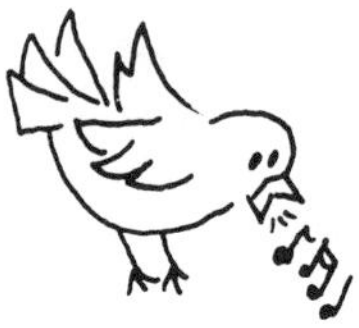

MAN-IN-THE-MOON CAKE

2–22A

1. Grate 1/4 cup lowfat cheese onto rice cake.

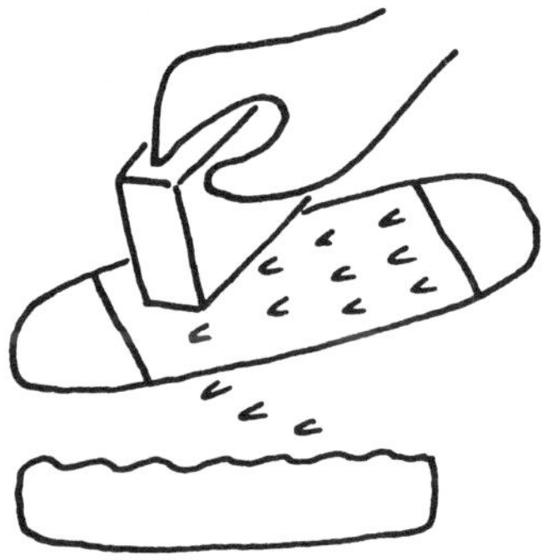

2. Put rice cake on baking sheet.

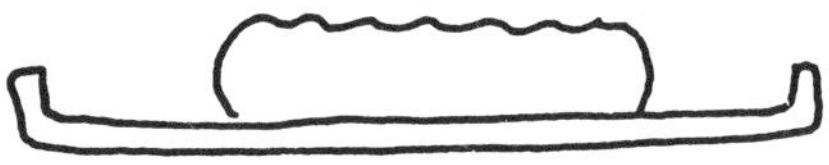

3. Broil in toaster oven until cheese melts.

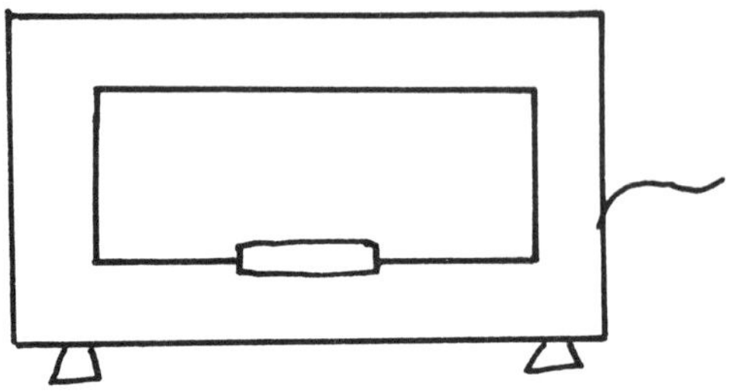

4. Put raisins on the cheese to make a face.

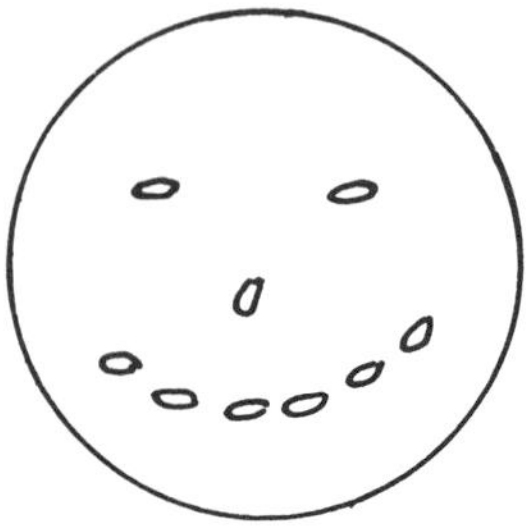

Name ____________________ Date ____________

STACKER CRACKERS

2–23A

1. Spread peanut butter on a cracker.

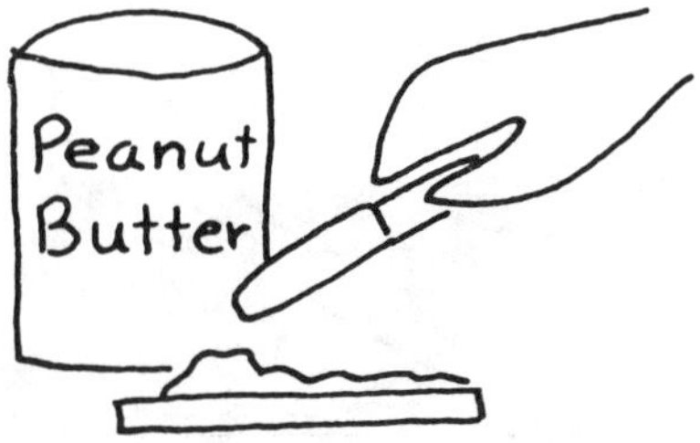

2. Cut 2 banana slices. Put them on the peanut butter.

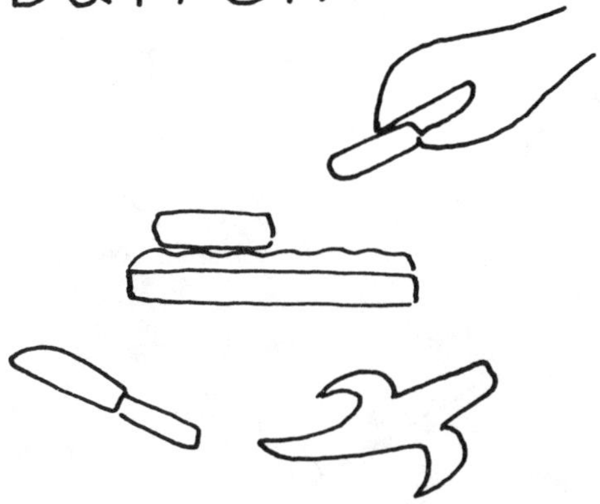

3. Put on another cracker, more peanut butter, and 2 more banana slices.

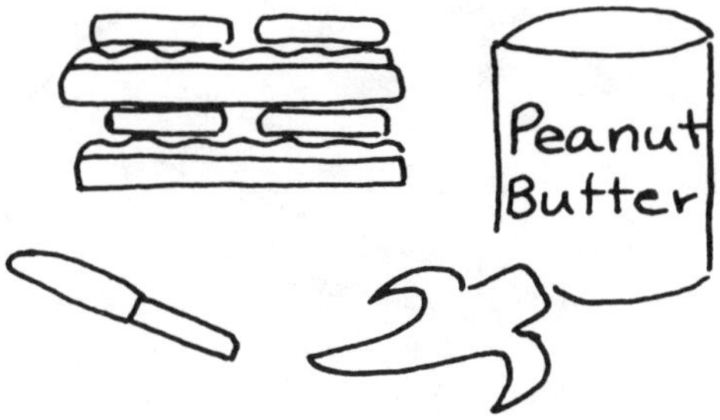

4. Put another cracker on top.

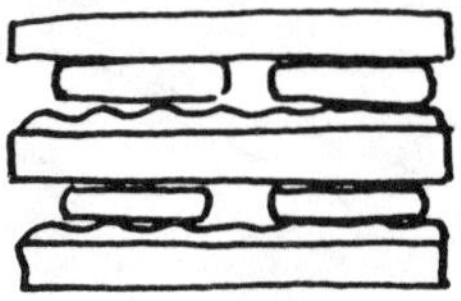

Name ______________________ Date ______________

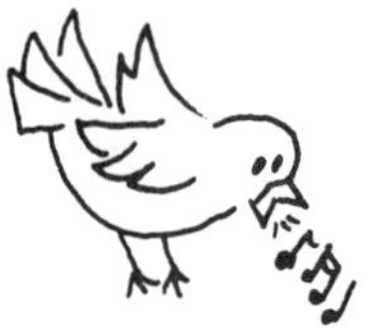

TURKEY ROLLAROUND

2–25A

1. Lay a carrot on a cheese slice. Roll the cheese around the carrot.

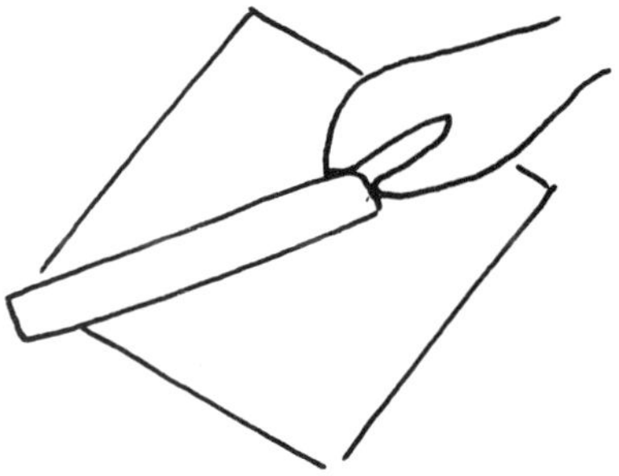

2. Spread mayonnaise on a turkey slice.

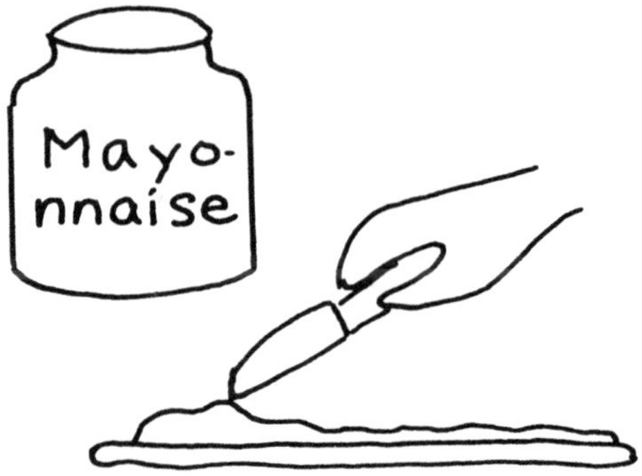

3. Roll the turkey around the cheese.

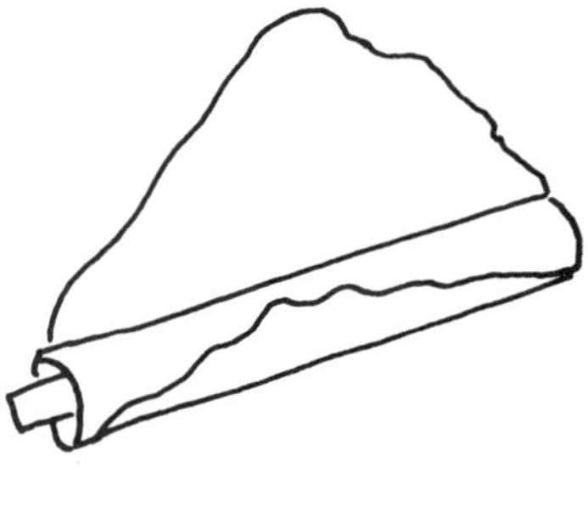

4. Roll a lettuce leaf around the turkey.

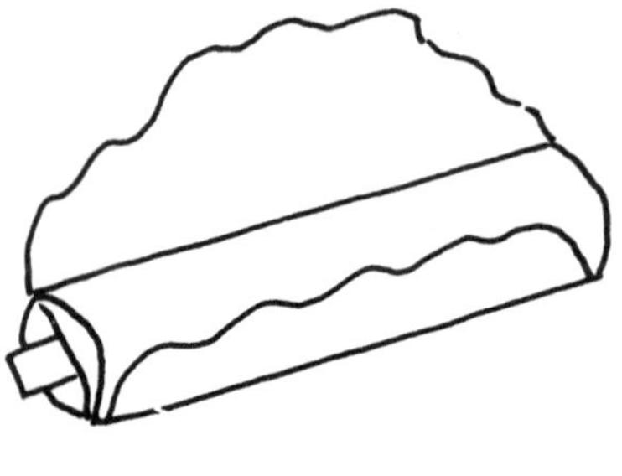

Name ______________________ Date ______________

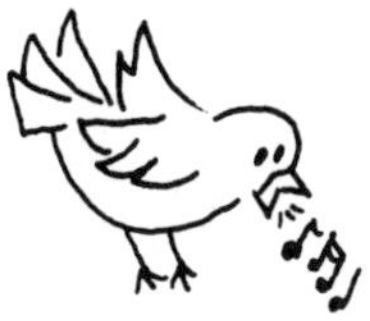

MINI-MUFFIN PIZZA *2–26A*

1. Spread tomato sauce on an English muffin half.

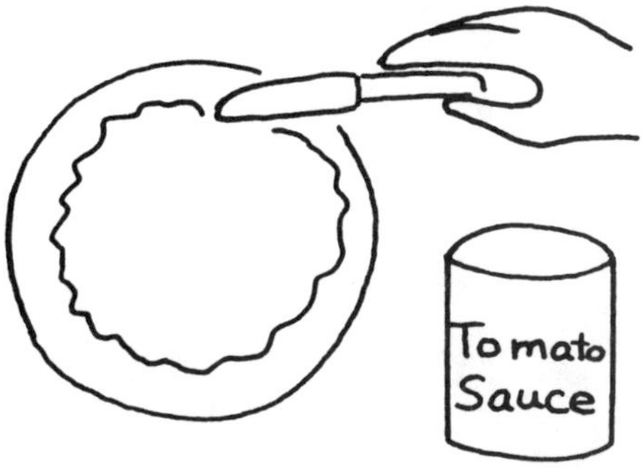

2. Grate 1/4 cup lowfat cheese onto tomato sauce.

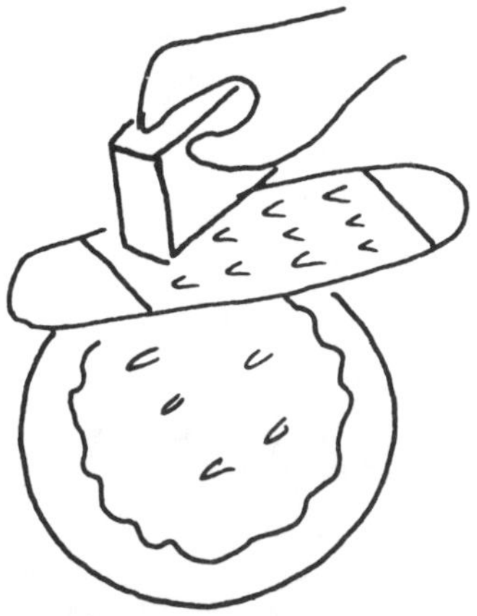

3. Put chopped mushrooms and green peppers on the cheese.

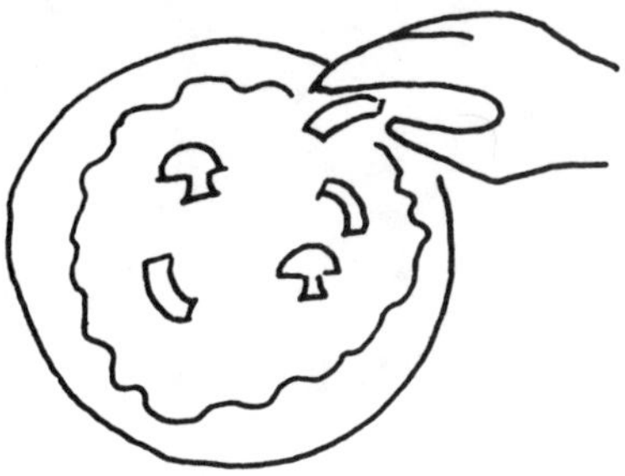

4. Broil in toaster oven until cheese melts.

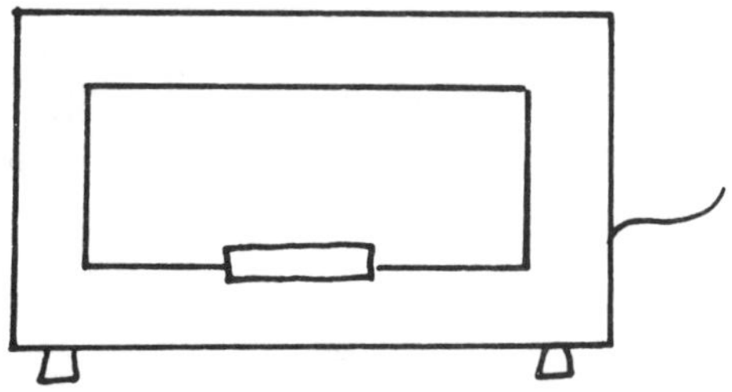

3 — *HEALTH HABITS*

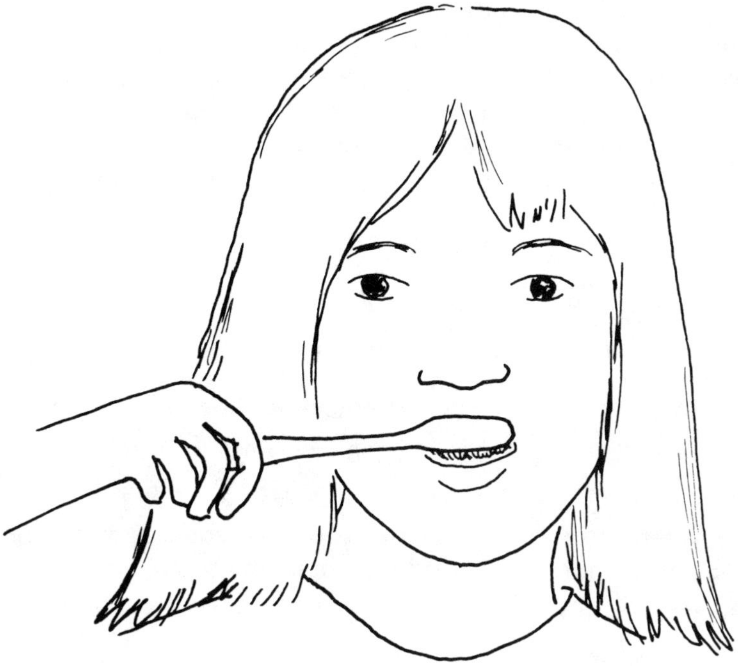

Children from four to eight years old are capable of learning and taking responsibility for many everyday health routines such as bathing, toothbrushing, hair grooming, hand washing, and dressing appropriately. By helping students develop good health habits now, you can influence the quality of their health and their lives in the future.

According to medical experts, most germs are spread hand-to-hand. For this reason, hand washing is perhaps the most important health habit for children to learn. Hand washing and other health habits tend to become automatic after they are practiced for several weeks. Emphasizing good health habits in the classroom will help students make them part of their daily routines. Your example can have an important effect, too, since young children learn by imitating the actions of others.

Many young children are fearful and anxious about visits to the doctor, dentist, health clinic, or hospital. Some of the activities in this section are designed to help students overcome those fears. Role playing is an important tool in helping young children become comfortable with unfamiliar situations. Allow ample time for students to act out health care situations and their anxieties about them.

Several review sheets are included in this section which reinforce information about good health habits which were introduced in earlier activities. These sheets may be used for review, as independent activities, or they may be placed in learning centers.

The activities in the Health Habits section will help students:

- learn about specific ways they can keep themselves healthy;
- understand the relationship between everyday actions and good health;
- establish health habits that will prevent the spread of germs;
- become familiar with and practice everyday routines such as bathing, toothbrushing, hair grooming, hand washing, and choosing appropriate clothing;
- become acquainted and comfortable with health care professionals, and find out how they help people stay healthy.

3–1 TAKE CARE OF YOUR TEETH

Help students learn how to have a healthy smile.

Materials:

chair	copies of Toothbrushing Chart 3–1A
towel	dental floss
small mirror	old dental X-rays
small table	dental equipment
several men's white shirts	toothbrush

Preparation:

1. Make arrangements for students to visit a nearby dental office. If this isn't possible, provide books about visiting the dentist. See Resource List for suggestions.
2. Set up a make-believe dental office in the classroom by covering a small table with a towel and placing a chair beside it. Put the mirror, X-rays, and dental equipment on the table.

Directions:

Take your students to the dental office at the time you have arranged. When you arrive, introduce them to the dentist, the dental assistant, the hygienist, and other staff members. Let the children take turns sitting in the examining chair. Ask the dentist to explain the basics of good dental care, and to demonstrate how to brush and floss teeth properly. If possible, let the children examine some of the equipment the dentist uses. Ask the dental assistant, the hygienist, and other staff members to briefly explain how they help people care for their teeth.

In the classroom, let the children take turns sitting in the chair and pretending to be dental patients. Have other students put on white shirts, buttoned in back, over their clothes and pretend to be the dentist, the dental assistant, and the hygienist.

Encourage the children to act out what they observed during their visit to the dental office, or in the books about visiting the dentist. For example, the dentist might look in the patient's mouth, consult the X-rays, and pretend to fill cavities. The dental assistant might count the patient's teeth and pretend to take X-rays.

Stress the importance of brushing teeth at least two times a day. Use a toothbrush to demonstrate correct brushing techniques. For front teeth, hold the brush at an angle so the bristles point toward the gumline. Then brush with a circular motion. For the inside and outside of back teeth, use short strokes with the brush at an angle. Then place the bristles flat on the chewing surfaces of the back teeth and scrub back and forth. Also explain how to floss teeth. Have the children pantomime the motions as you demonstrate them.

Distribute the Toothbrushing Charts and have students add them to their "Here's to My Health" booklet file folders. Encourage students to color a space on their charts each morning and evening after they brush their teeth.

3–2 GLAD TEETH, SAD TEETH

Help students learn which foods build strong teeth and which foods cause decay.

Materials:

old magazines
copies of Food Picture page 1–2B
copies of Glad Tooth and Sad Tooth activity sheets 3–2A and 3–2B
crayons
scissors
glue

Preparation:

1. Cut out magazine pictures of Milk Group foods such as milk, cheese, and others.
2. Cut out magazine pictures of candy, ice cream, and other sugary snacks.

Directions:

Discuss with students the foods that build strong teeth and bones (foods from the Milk Group). Also talk about foods that weaken teeth and cause decay (candy, ice cream, sugary snacks). Show magazine pictures of each type of food.

Distribute a Food Picture page, a Glad Tooth activity sheet, and a Sad Tooth activity sheet to each student. Have students color the foods on their Food Picture pages, and then cut on the lines to make twelve individual food pictures. Ask them to classify the food pictures by gluing those that help build strong teeth to their Glad Tooth activity sheets, and those that weaken teeth and cause decay to their Sad Tooth activity sheets.

3–3 VISITING THE DOCTOR

Help students understand how doctors and other medical professionals help them stay well.

Materials:

low table
butcher or mural paper
masking tape
dolls
some of the following equipment and supplies:

stethoscopes	disposable plastic syringes, without needles
lightweight rubber gloves	small medicine droppers
gauze pads, cotton balls	face masks

Preparation:

1. Make arrangements for students to visit a nearby medical office or hospital. If this isn't possible, provide books about visiting the doctor. See Resource List for suggestions.
2. Set up a make-believe medical office in the classroom by taping butcher or mural paper over a low table to serve as an examining table. Place medical equipment and supplies nearby.

Directions:

Take your students to the medical office or hospital at the time you have arranged, or read aloud books about visiting the doctor. Discuss ways doctors, nurses, and other medical professionals help people stay healthy:

- Doctors and nurses care for people who are sick.
- Doctors prescribe medicines that help us get well.
- Doctors and nurses give injections that keep us from getting certain diseases.
- Doctors and nurses weigh, measure, and examine us to make sure we are strong and healthy.
- Doctors and nurses tell us about ways to stay healthy, such as being sure to get enough sleep, eat nutritious meals, and wash our hands before meals and after using the bathroom.

In the classroom, let the children take turns pretending to be doctors, nurses, and patients. Invite the patients to lie on the examining table while the doctors and nurses gently examine them. Some children may wish to pretend to be parents who are bringing their sick children (dolls) to the doctor. Encourage students to act out what they observed during their visit to the medical office, or in the books about visiting the doctor. Show how students can use a stethoscope to listen to a friend's heartbeat. Continue the activity until all of the students have had turns to use all of the equipment.

3–4 FIRST AID FACTS

Cuts and scrapes are part of every child's life. Here's how to care for them properly.

Materials:

copies of First Aid activity sheet 3–4A
small plastic bandages (optional)
crayons

Directions:

Talk with students about what to do when they get small cuts or scrapes while playing. Emphasize these steps in caring for minor injuries:

- Tell an adult what has happened.
- Press the cut with a clean cloth until it stops bleeding.
- Wash the cut carefully with soap and water.
- Gently dry it with a clean towel.
- Leave the cut open to the air, or cover it with a plastic bandage.

Distribute copies of the First Aid activity sheet. Ask students to draw faces and other details on the figures. Then tell them to pretend the child on the activity sheet has fallen and gotten hurt. Have students draw the imaginary wounds and put plastic bandages on them, or draw on bandages.

3–5 WASH, WASH, WASH YOUR HANDS

It is important for children to get into the handwashing habit.

Materials:

plastic basins or tubs
lukewarm water
soap
towels
copies of Wash, Wash, Wash Your Hands activity sheet 3–5A
scissors
glue

Directions:

Discuss handwashing with students and explain that washing our hands gets rid of harmful germs that can make us sick. Stress that students should always wash their hands before eating, after using the bathroom, after blowing their noses, and whenever their hands are dirty.

Fill several plastic basins or tubs with lukewarm water. Sing the following verse with the students to the tune of "Row, Row, Row Your Boat." Have students wash their hands with soap in the water, and then dry them on the towels while they sing. If it's not possible to use water, have students pantomime washing their hands. Afterwards, help students complete the Wash, Wash, Wash Your Hands activity sheets.

Wash, wash, wash your hands
Wash them every day.
Wash, wash, wash your hands
To keep the germs away.

3–6 HEALTHFUL HELPERS

Play a guessing game with students to help them discover healthful helpers for good grooming.

Materials:

copies of Healthful Helpers picture page 3–6A
crayons
scissors
glue
index cards
craft sticks

Directions:

Distribute the Healthful Helpers picture pages. Have students color the pictures, then cut them apart to make six individual pictures. Tell students to make six Healthful Helper signs by gluing each picture to an index card, and then gluing on craft stick handles.

When students have finished making their signs, read the following poem aloud. Ask students to decide which grooming aid each verse describes, and hold up that sign.

Use me in the shower.
Float me in the tub.
Put me on your wash cloth
And scrubba, scrubba, scrub. (soap)

Spread me on your toothbrush
Every single day.
Then brusha, brusha, brusha
Help keep cavities away. (toothpaste)

Use us every morning
When you get out of bed.
We'll take away the tangles
If you'll use us on your head. (comb and brush)

A piece of me between your teeth
Pulled gently to and fro.
Up and down, side to side
Helps the food to go. (dental floss)

When your hair is dirty
Rub me in your hair.
Rub-a-dub. Rub-a-dub.
Make some lather there.
Rub-a-dub. Rub-a-dub.
Rinse off the lather so
Your hair will be squeaky clean
With a healthy glow. (shampoo)

I'm soft, clean, and fluffy
So give me a try
After baths or showers
When it's time to dry. (towel)

3–7 WHAT GOES IN YOUR MOUTH?

Students can keep germs from spreading if they know what they should and shouldn't put in their mouths.

Materials:

copies of What Goes in Your Mouth? activity sheet 3–7A
crayons

Directions:

Ask students what they know about germs. After they give their ideas, explain that germs are so small we cannot see them, but they can still make us sick. Help students understand that germs are all around us but we can help keep germs out of our bodies by putting only clean things into our mouths. Read the following list aloud and ask students to clap when they hear the name of something that is all right to put in their mouths. Afterwards, ask what is the same about those things. (They are all foods or other clean objects that are free of germs.)

apple	cracker	marker
pencil	shoelace	sponge
rubber band	necklace	cup
toothbrush	cheese slice	cookie
fork	carrot	hairbrush
scissors	toy car	barrette
fingers	chopsticks	banana

Distribute the What Goes In Your Mouth? activity sheets. Help students read the directions and complete the sheet.

3–8 SKIN PROTECTION

It is important for children to learn to avoid sunburn.

Materials:

bottle of sunscreen (optional)
copies of Skin Protection activity sheet 3–8A
crayons

Directions:

Ask students to tell about times when they have been out in the sun for a long time such as going to the beach, spending the day at the park, or going for a boat ride. After they describe their experiences, explain that it is important to keep their skin from being burned by the hot rays of the sun. If possible, show the bottle of sunscreen, pass it around, and let the students take off the cap to look at and smell it. Tell students that they should rub sunscreen onto any areas of skin that will be exposed to the sun for a long time. Mention that hats, long sleeved shirts, and other types of clothing can also protect skin from the sun.

Lead the children in pantomiming how they might get ready for a day at the park. Be sure to include putting on a hat, sunglasses, and sunscreen.

Distribute the Skin Protection activity sheets. Help students read the directions and complete the sheet.

3–9 BATH TIME

Use dolls to help students practice good grooming habits.

Materials:

- plastic basins or water table
- lukewarm water
- soap
- shampoo
- sponges or washcloths
- towels
- washable dolls and clothes
- combs or hairbrushes

Preparation:

1. Send home notes asking each child to bring in a washable doll.
2. Fill the plastic basins or water table with lukewarm water.

Directions:

Let the students take turns bathing their dolls in the basins of water. Emphasize that it is important to wash every body part thoroughly. After the baths, suggest that the children also wash the dolls' hair. Encourage the children to talk about their own bathtime routines.

Have the children use the towels to thoroughly dry the dolls and their hair. After the dolls are dressed, suggest that the students play barber or beauty shop by combing and styling the dolls' hair, and pretending to cut it with imaginary scissors.

3–10 WAKE UP, SLEEPYHEAD

Tell students that getting enough sleep is important for good health. Ask them to tell what time they go to bed at night and what time they get up in the morning. Then discuss these sleep concepts with the group:

- Your body grows while you are asleep.
- Your body builds up energy while you are asleep.
- People become cross and grouchy if they don't get enough sleep.
- People who are tired are more likely to get sick.
- Sleep gives your heart the rest it needs.
- Children four to eight years old need ten to twelve hours of sleep each night.

Read the poem aloud, and have the children act out the motions:

Daytime is over.
It's time for bed.
Pajamas on now,
Sleepyhead.
Pull down the shades.
Hug teddy bear tight.
Fold down the covers.
Turn on the night light.
Brush your teeth and
Wash hands and face,
Then climb into
Your resting place.

Wake up. Wake up,
Sleepyhead.
Yawn and stretch.
Get out of bed.
Wash face and hands.
Comb your hair.
Brush your teeth
And dress with care.
Look in the mirror.
Smile and say,
"Today I'll have
A special day."

3–11 AH-CHOO!

People who have colds often cough and sneeze, spreading their cold germs to others.

Materials:

drawing paper
scissors
crayons
glue
tissues

Directions:

Have the students each draw a picture of their face on drawing paper and color it. Ask them to trace around their hands, then color and cut out the hands. Help students glue a crumpled tissue near the mouth on their faces, and then glue the hand cutout over the tissue.

Discuss with students what to do when they have a cold. Emphasize the value of helping the body build up a resistance to colds by:

- a healthy diet
- cleanliness
- exercise
- rest
- plenty of fluids
- staying away from others with colds.

Read the poems aloud and have students act out the motions:

Please cover your mouth
With a tissue or two
If you have to cough
Or sneeze an "AH-CHOO!"
Please toss them away
After one sneeze and blow
Then wash hands and dry them
So cold germs will go.

When you have a cold
In your chest or head
Put on pajamas
And climb into bed.
Pull up the covers
And snuggle down deep
Drink lots of juices
And get plenty of sleep.

Have students hold up their pictures to share.

3–12 HEIGHT AND WEIGHT

A child's height and weight are indicators of his or her general health. Help students learn how to record these statistics.

Materials:

yardstick or tape measure
copies of Watch Me Grow! chart 3–12A
long sheet of butcher or mural paper
masking tape
bathroom scale
markers

Preparation:

Tape the butcher or mural paper vertically to a wall.

Directions:

Introduce the word *height* and explain that it is the distance, measured in units called inches, from the top of a person's head to the bottom of his or her feet. Have students take turns standing with their backs against the butcher paper while a friend marks where the top of each one's head comes. Then help each student use a yardstick or tape measure to find out how many inches tall he or she is. Distribute the Watch Me Grow! charts and help students record their heights.

Introduce the word *weight* and explain that we measure how heavy people are in units called pounds. Read the following poem aloud and have students do as it says:

Take off your shoes.
Wiggle your toes.
Step on the scale awhile.
Hold very still.
Don't jiggle all
The numbers on the dial.

Gain or lose
A pound, an ounce
You're growing day by day.
The scale helps you
Figure it out
So write down what you weigh.

Help students record their weights on their Watch Me Grow! charts. Then have them add the charts to their "Here's to My Health" booklet file folders. Encourage them to continue to measure and record their height and weight each month at home.

3–13 DRESS FOR THE WEATHER

Dressing properly for different kinds of weather helps people stay healthy.

Materials:

flannelboard
Dress for the Weather patterns 3–13A and 3–13B
felt squares

Preparation:

1. Use the Dress for the Weather patterns to cut flannelboard figures from felt.

Directions:

Talk with the children about why we wear different types of clothing in hot, cold, rainy, and windy weather. Help them understand that clothing protects their bodies, keeping them warm in cold weather or cool in hot weather. Then have them suggest what to wear on a hot day, a snowy day, a rainy day, and a windy day.

Place the felt child figure on the flannelboard and put the other felt cutouts nearby. Then read the following poem aloud. After verses 2, 3, 4, and 5, ask a child to come to the flannelboard, pick out the clothes that would be best for the type of weather described, and "dress" the felt child figure in them.

1. Check the weather report
Early each day
To dress for the weather
In the right way.

2. It's snowy and icy.
It's cold and gray.
How should you dress
On a cold weather day?

3. It's humid and hot.
There's lots of sun.
How should you dress
For hot weather fun?

4. It's rainy and splashy
With puddles about.
How should you dress
When rain clouds are out?

5. It's warmish and nice
Then turns breezy cool.
How should you dress
When you head for school?

3–14 HEALTH HABIT GAMES

These activities can help your students remember ways to care for their health.

MATCH-UPS

Materials:

comb	shampoo
brush	towel
washcloth	adhesive cream
bar of soap	plastic bandage
toothbrush	emery board
toothpaste	nailbrush

Directions:

Spread out all the items on the table. Move them around and mix them up so that items that are used together are not next to each other. Have students take turns picking out two items that are used together, naming them, and then pantomiming how they are used.

WHAT IS IT?

Materials:

box with lid (approximately 12″ square)
gift wrapping paper, tape (optional)
Health care items from *Match-Ups* activity

Preparation:

1. Cut a 4″ square opening in the lid of the box.
2. Place the health care items in the box.
3. If you wish, cover the box and lid with gift wrapping paper.

Directions:

Have students take turns reaching into the box, through the hole in the lid, and feeling one object. Before removing the object, ask each student to describe what he or she is touching and then guess what it is. Then have the student take the object out, show it to the class, and explain how it is used to keep people healthy.

SING-ALONG

Sing the following verse, to the tune of "Here We Go Round the Mulberry Bush," with students. Ask them to act out the health habits described in each verse as they sing.

This is the way I wash my face,
Wash my face, wash my face.
This is the way I wash my face
So early in the morning.

Ask students to suggest other health habits to sing about in the song. Some possibilities are "brush my teeth," "comb my hair," and "wash my hair." Repeat the song, using students' suggestions.

GOOD HEALTH HABITS

Good health habits learned at an early age will stay with a child for life.

Discuss how exercising, getting enough rest, and proper eating are some good health habits to learn. Mention that it is important to drink several glasses of water every day. Ask students to think of other good health habits they have learned.

Have the students form a large circle. Start the group clapping as you read the poem aloud, using the name of the child on your right. After the verse, ask that student to tell a good health habit. Continue to chant the verse until each child has had a turn.

Justin, Justin, won't you tell
A good health habit to keep you well.

Maria, Maria, won't you tell
A good health habit to keep you well.

3–15 HEALTH HABITS REVIEW SHEETS

This is a good time to review what the children have learned about health habits.

Materials:

copies of review sheets 3–15A through 3–15F
pencils

Directions:

Have copies of these review sheets available. They may be used for review, as independent activities, or they may be placed in learning centers.

Activity Sheets for Section 3: Health Habits

3–1A	Toothbrushing Chart
3–2A	Glad Tooth
3–2B	Sad Tooth
3–4A	First Aid
3–5A	Wash, Wash, Wash Your Hands
3–6A	Healthful Helpers
3–7A	What Goes in Your Mouth?
3–8A	Skin Protection
3–12A	Watch Me Grow!
3–13A	Dress for the Weather
3–13B	Dress for the Weather
3–15A	Health Hint
3–15B	Health Scramble
3–15C	Who Is It?
3–15D	Take Care of Your Health
3–15E	Take Care of Your Health
3–15F	Good Grooming

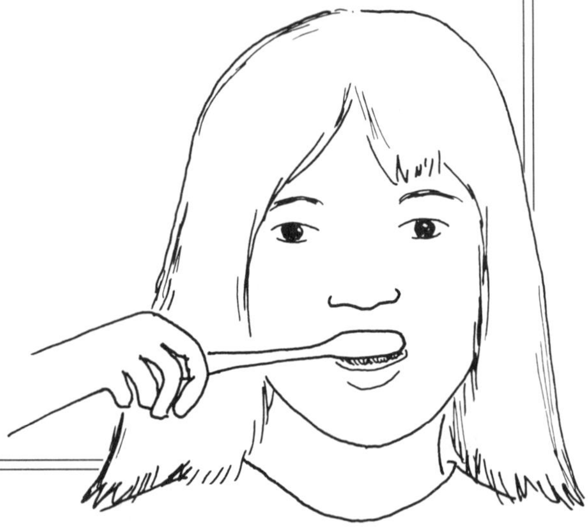

Name ______________________ **Date** ______________________

TOOTHBRUSHING CHART 3–1A

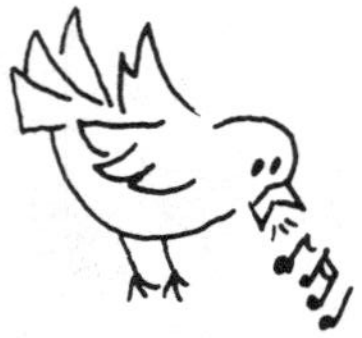

Brush your teeth two times a day.

Color a space each time you brush.

Week 1	Mon.	Tues.	Wed.	Thurs.	Fri.	Sat.	Sun.
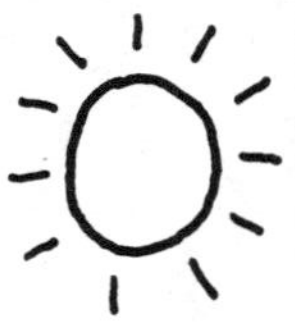							

Week 2	Mon.	Tues.	Wed.	Thurs.	Fri.	Sat.	Sun.
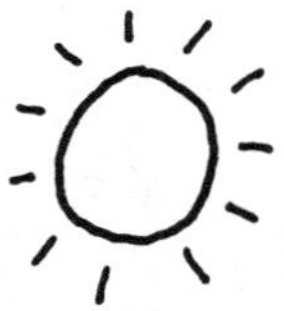							

Name ______________________ Date ______________

GLAD TOOTH

3–2A

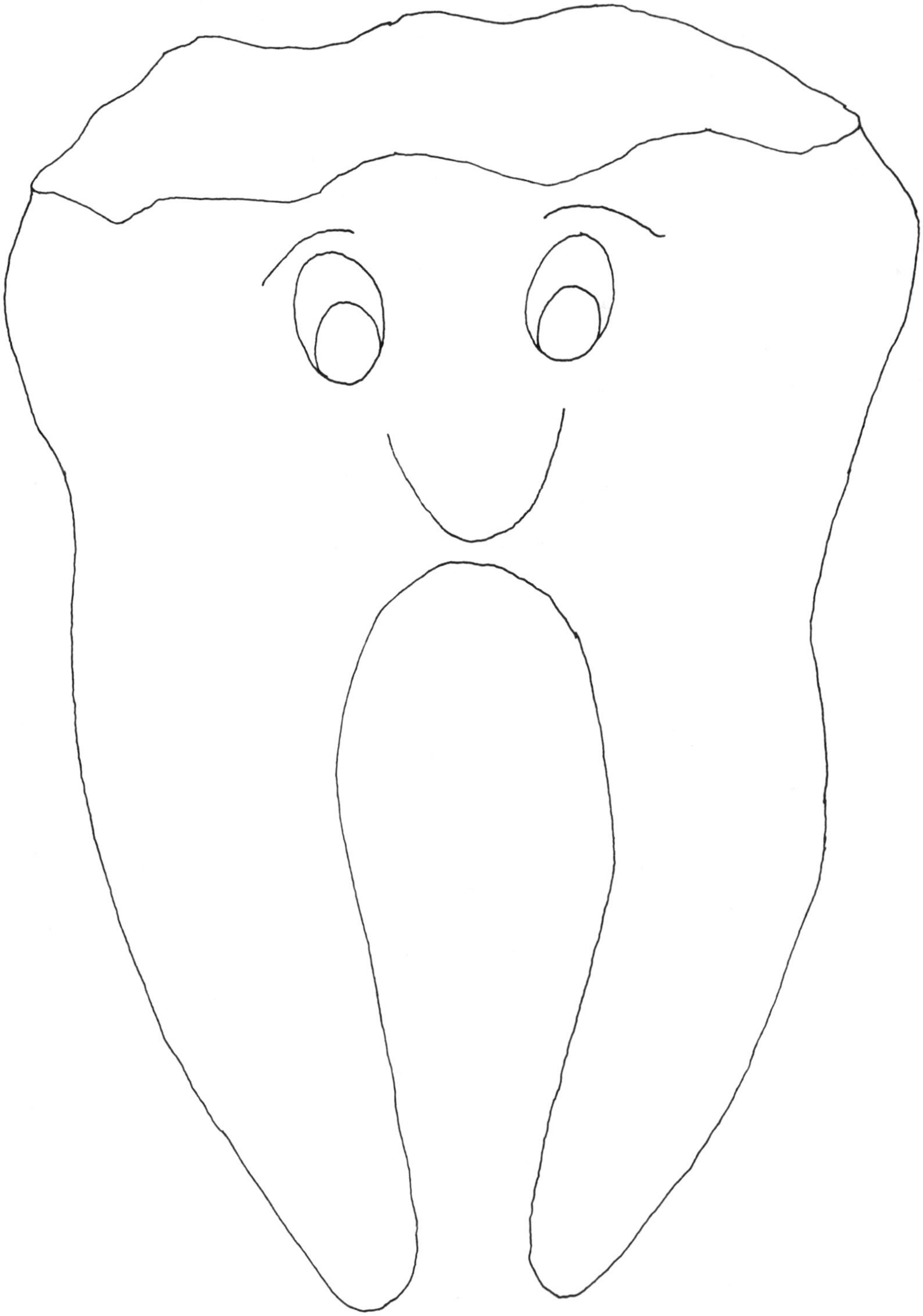

Name ____________________ Date ____________

SAD TOOTH

3–2B

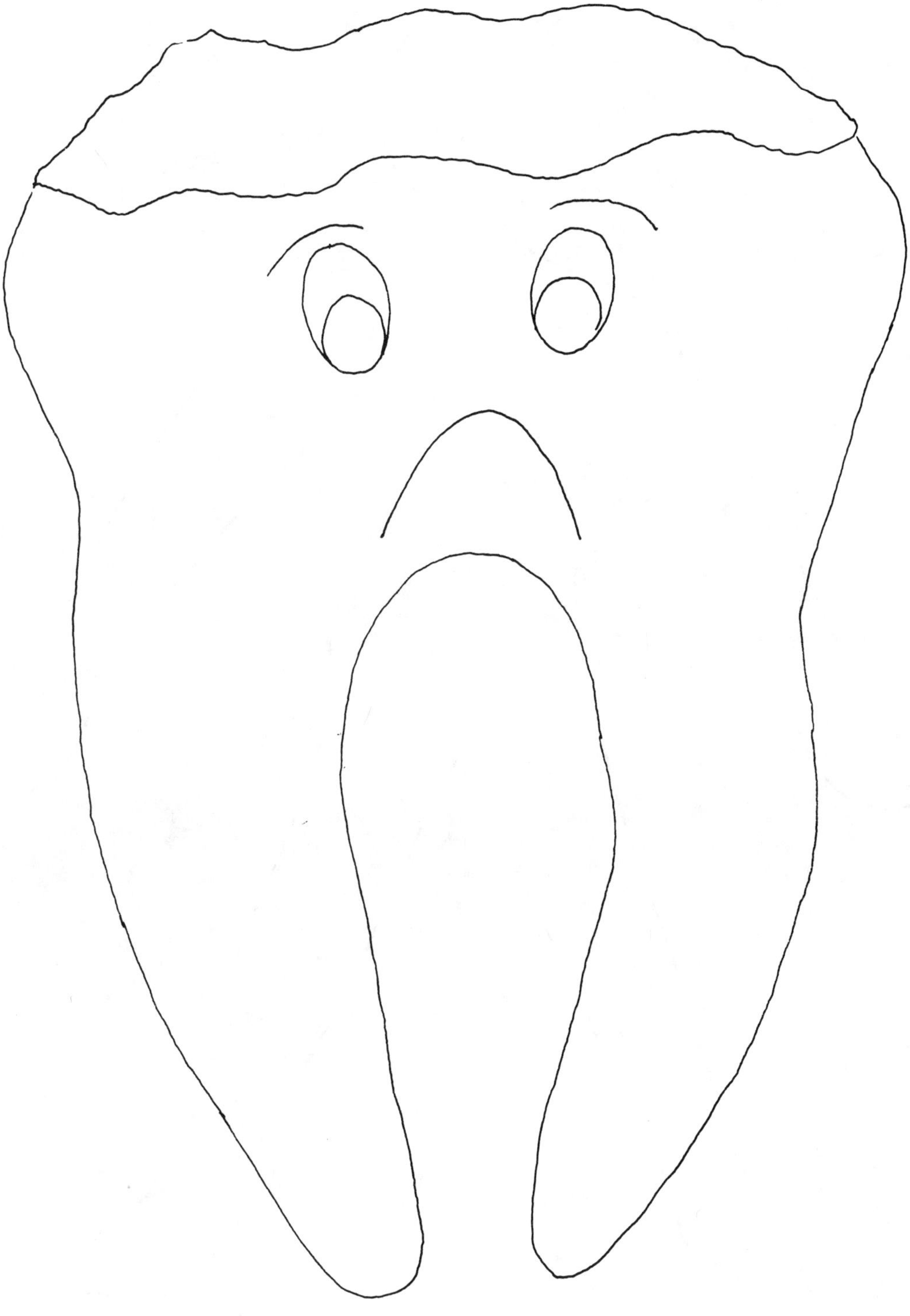

Name ______________________________ Date ________________

FIRST AID *3–4A*

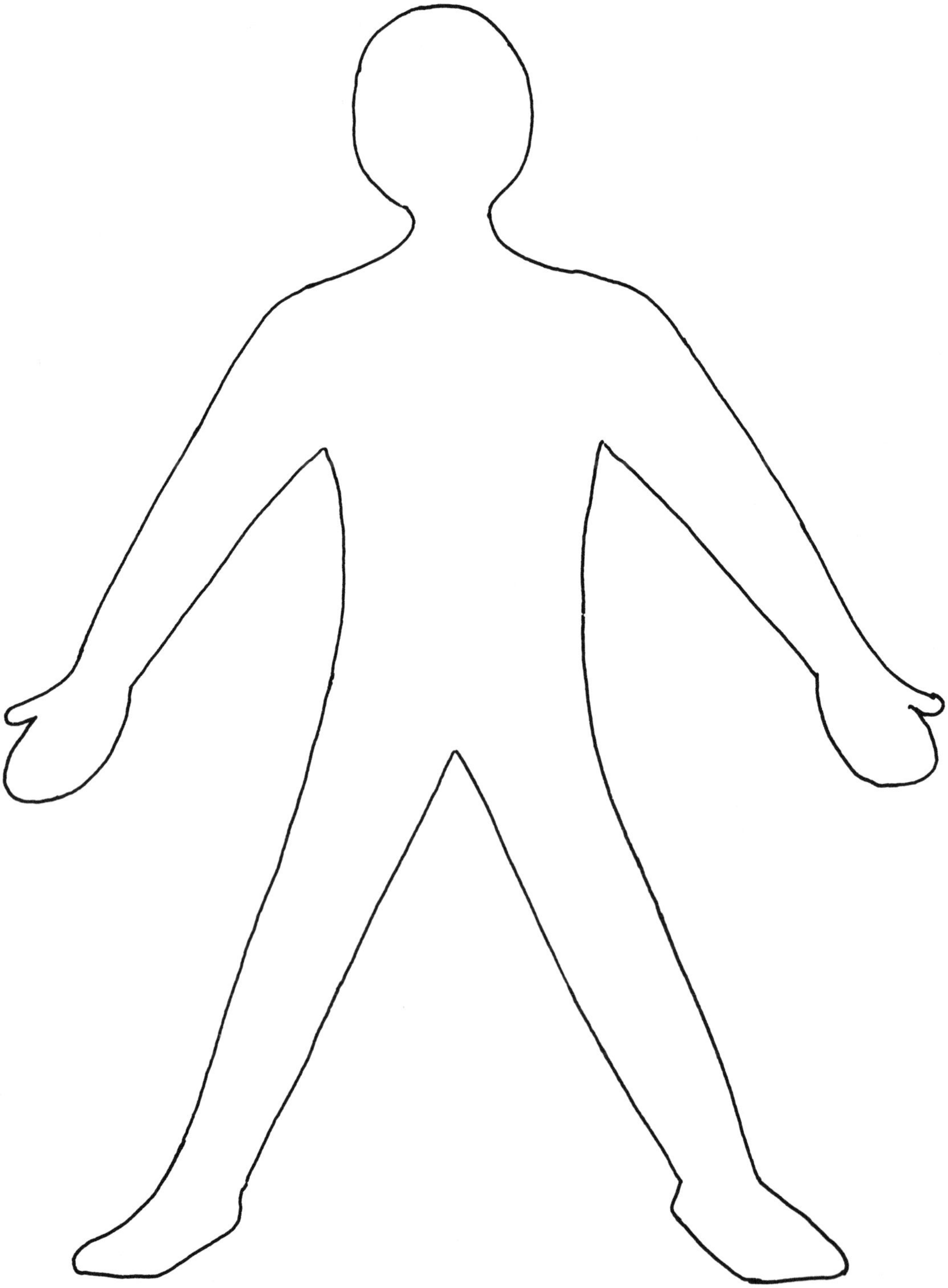

Name ______________________ Date ______________

WASH, WASH, WASH YOUR HANDS *3–5A*

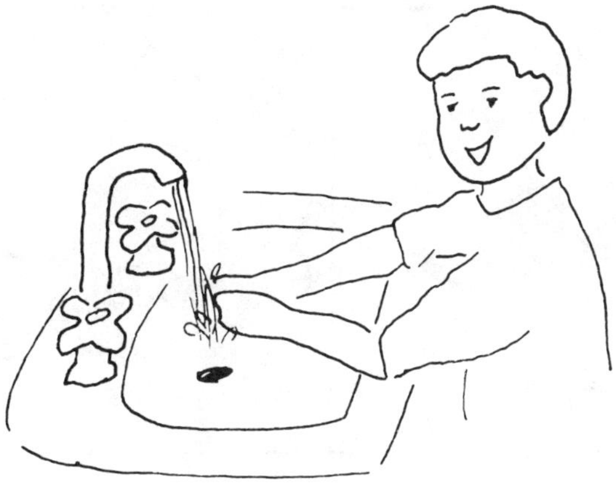

Cut out the words below. Paste them in the blanks to show when you should wash your hands.

Wash Your Hands:

Before you _ _ _ .

After using the _ _ _ _ _ _ _ _ .

When your hands are _ _ _ _ _ .

After blowing your _ _ _ _ .

nose	bathroom
dirty	eat

Name ______________________________ Date ________________

HEALTHFUL HELPERS *3–6A*

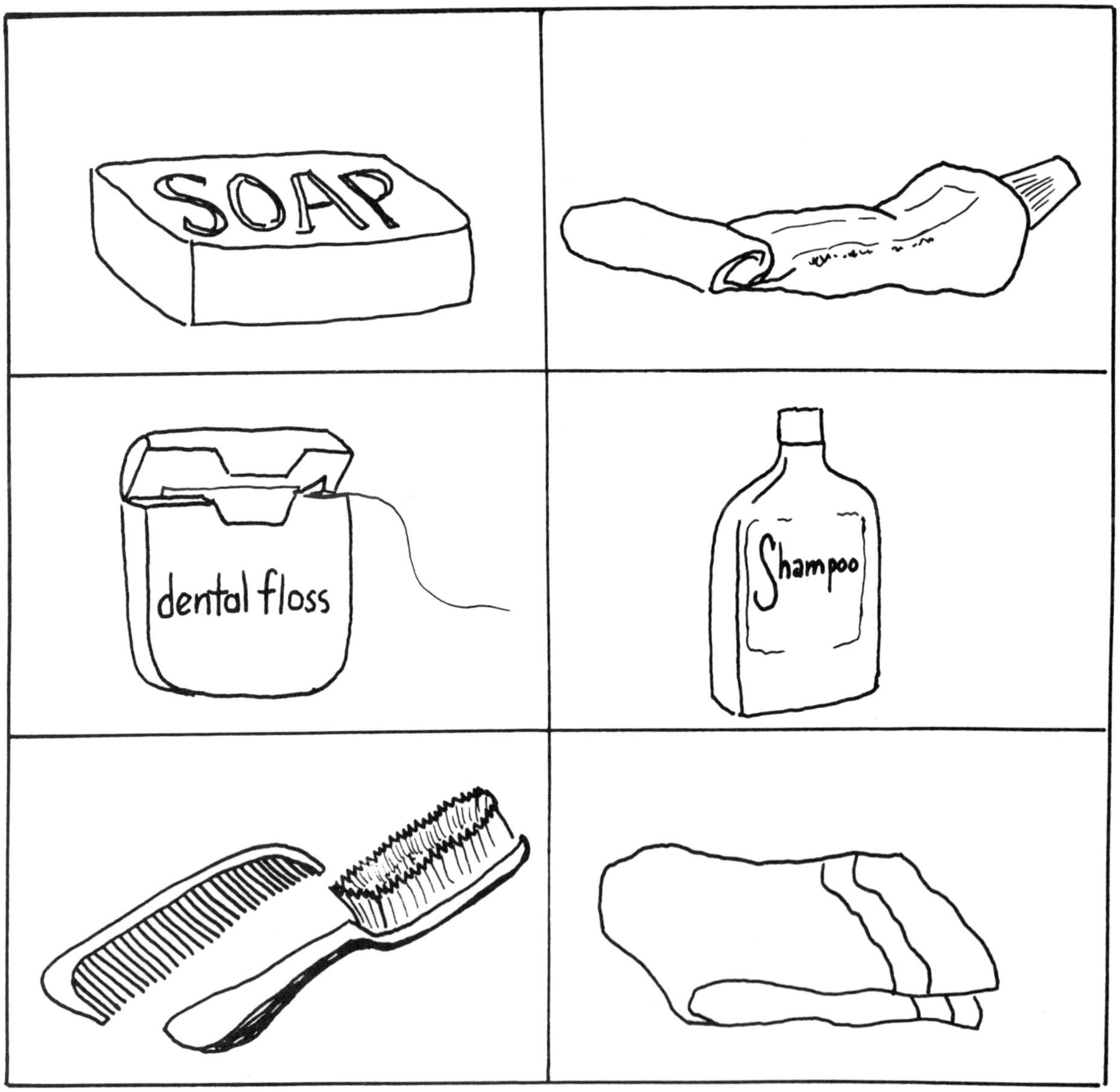

Name ______________________________ **Date** ______________

WHAT GOES IN YOUR MOUTH? *3–7A*

Color the items that are all right to put in your mouth. Put an X on the ones you should not put in your mouth.

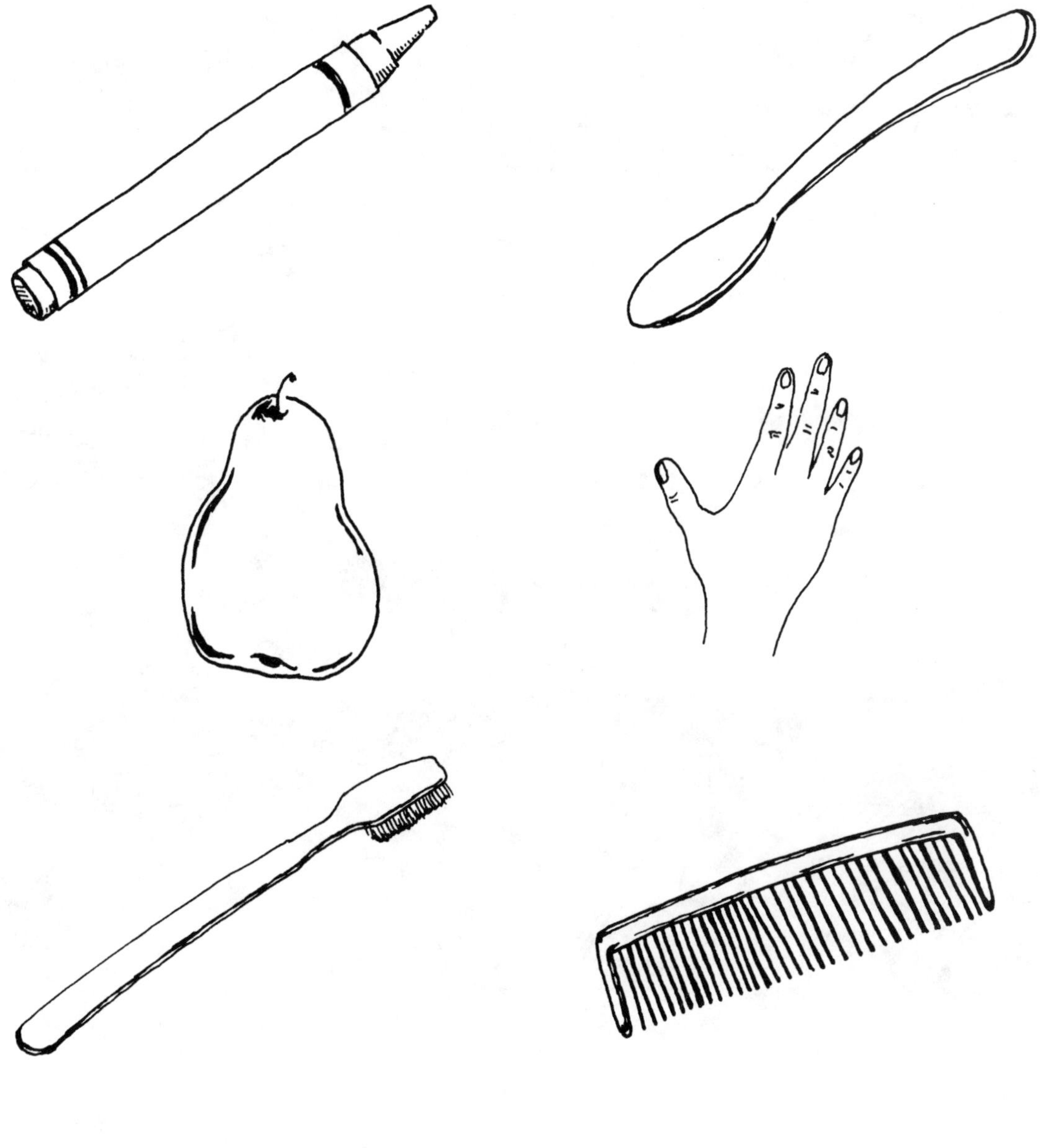

Name ______________________ Date ______________

SKIN PROTECTION *3–8A*

Remember to protect your skin when you are out in the sun. Circle the things that protect you from the sun. Color the picture.

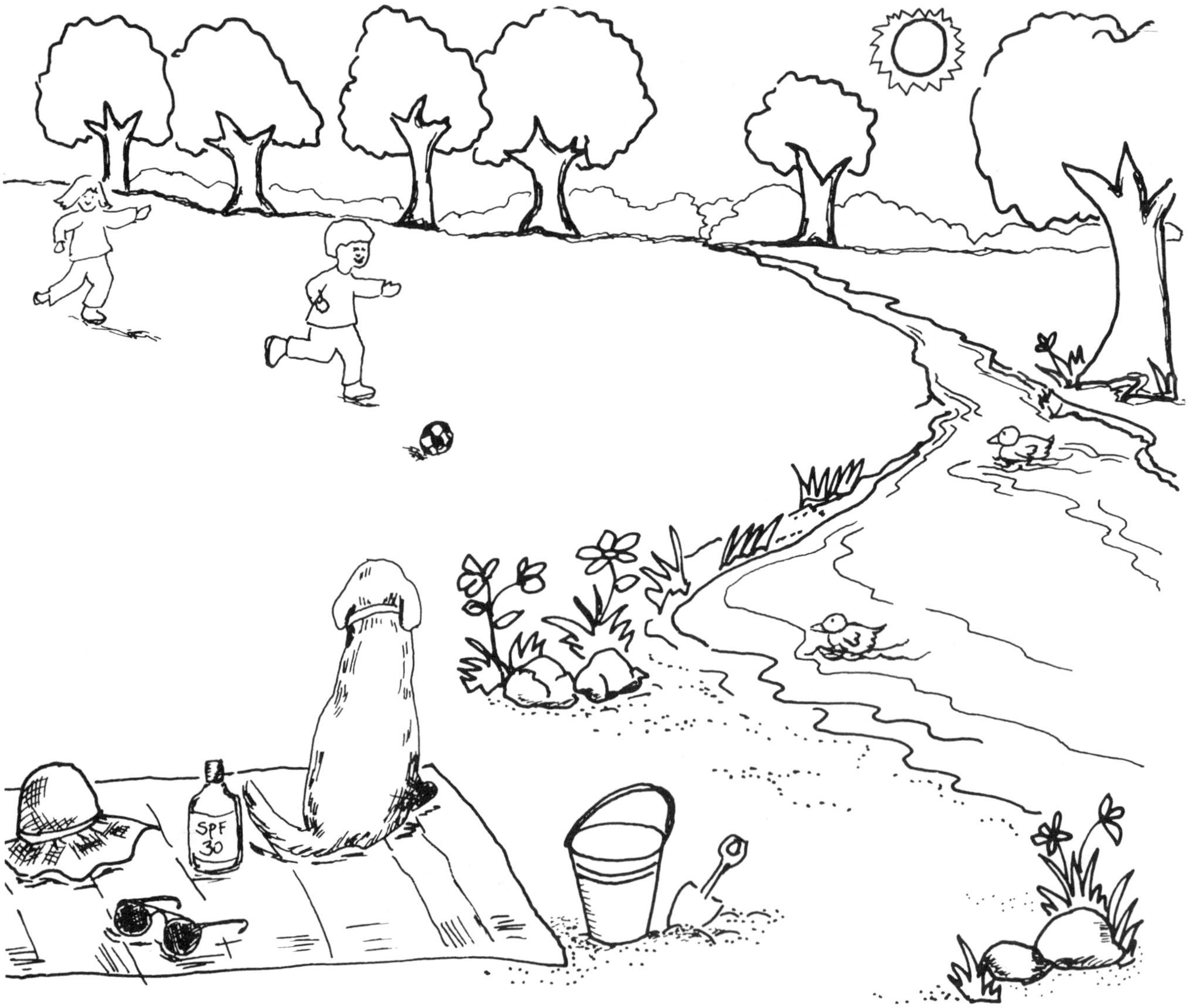

Name ______________________________ Date ________________

WATCH ME GROW! 3–12A

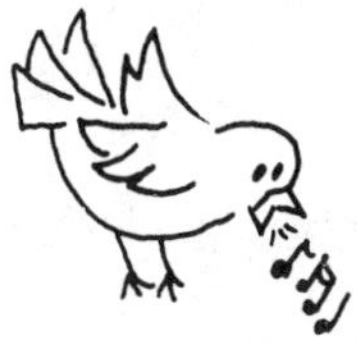

Watch Me Grow!

	Height	Weight
September	____ inches	____ pounds
October	____	____
November	____	____
December	____	____
January	____	____
February	____	____
March	____	____
April	____	____
May	____	____
June	____	____

Name ______________________ Date ______________________

DRESS FOR THE WEATHER *3–13A*

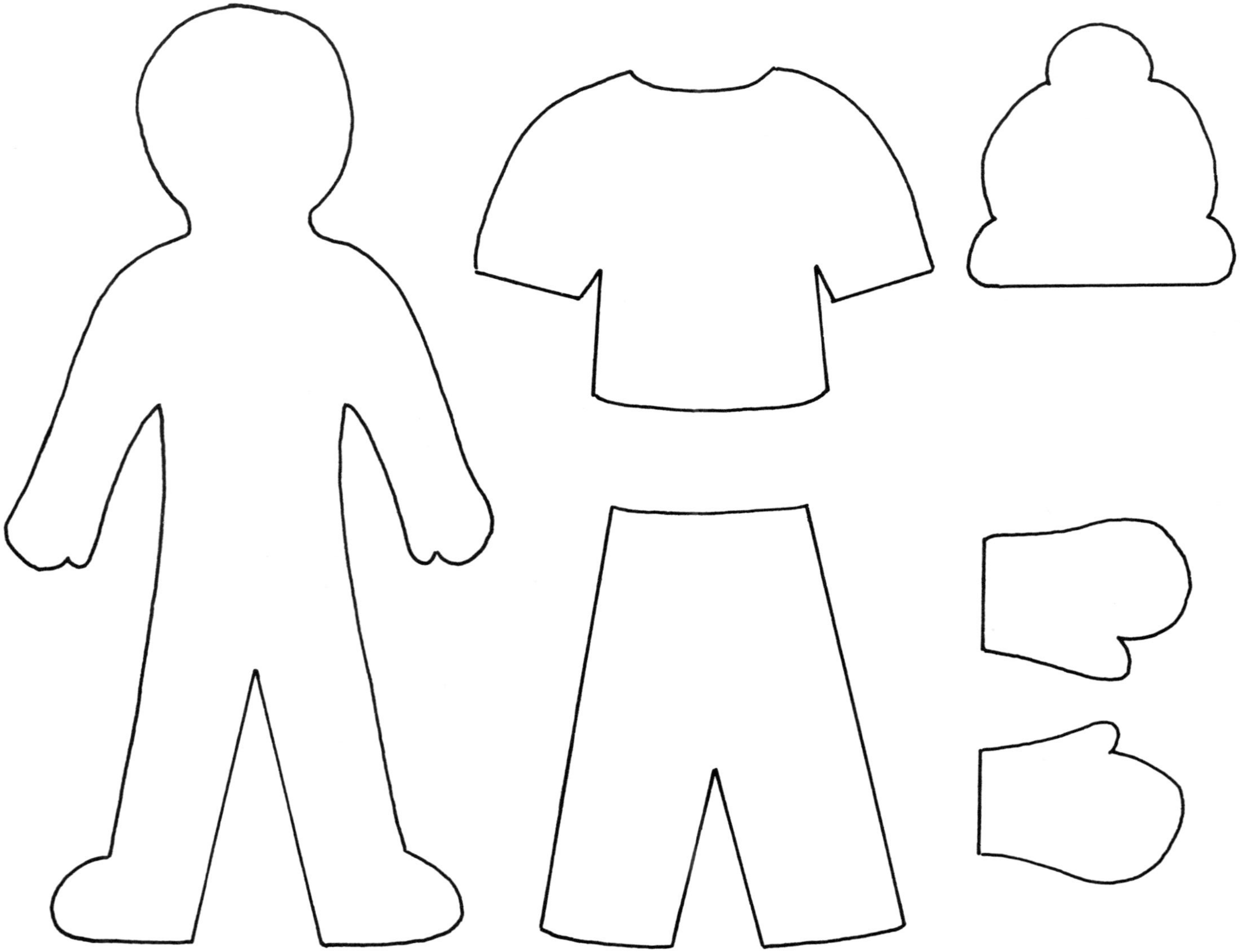

Name ______________________ **Date** ______________________

DRESS FOR THE WEATHER *3–13B*

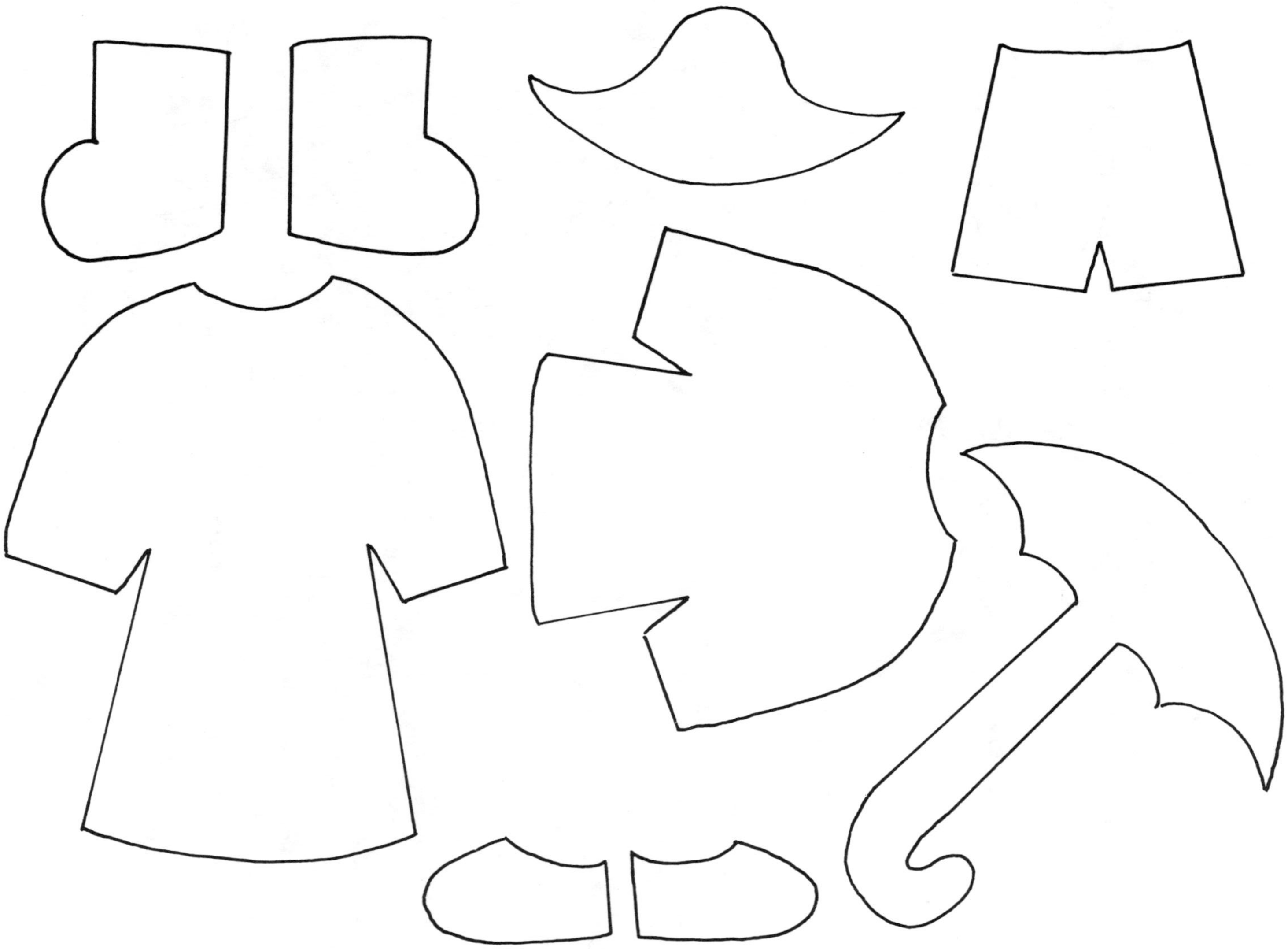

Name ______________________ Date ______________

HEALTH HINT

3–15A

This health hint tells something you should do every day. Start at the arrow. Circle the first letter and then every other letter until you come to the exclamation point. Write the circled letters in the spaces below the glass.

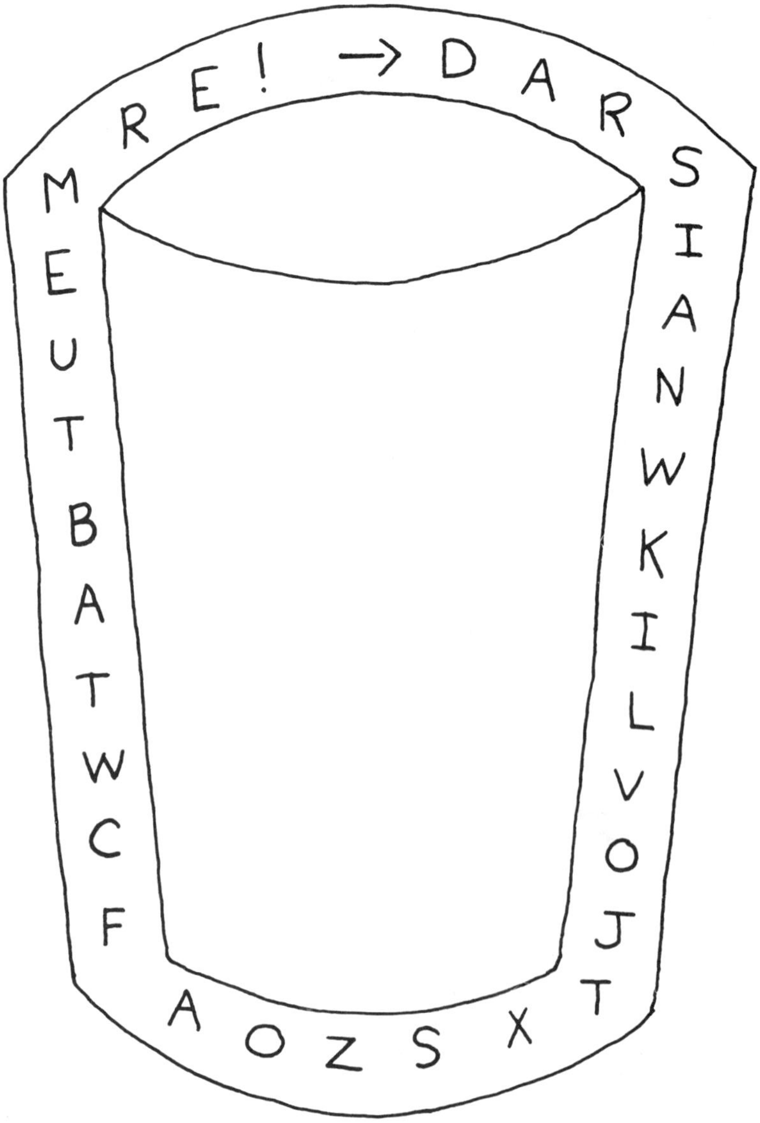

_ _ _ _ _   _ _ _ _   _ _   _ _ _ _ _ _!

Name ______________________ Date ______________

HEALTH SCRAMBLE *3–15B*

Unscramble the words below each question. Write the words in the blanks to answer the questions.

1. What should you always do before you eat?
   SHAW ORUY SHDNA

   ____

2. What is one way to keep your teeth healthy?
   SHRUB OWT MITES A DYA

   ____

   ____

3. What do you need every day?
   EECEISRX

   ____

4. What do you need every night?
   NET RUSOH OF PLESE

   ____

   ____

Name ______________________________ Date ________________

WHO IS IT? *3–15C*

Cut out and paste the pictures in the spaces to answer the questions.

1. Who keeps your teeth clean and healthy?

2. Who helps you feel better when you are sick?

3. Who takes care of you at home?

4. Who weighs and measures you at the doctor's office?

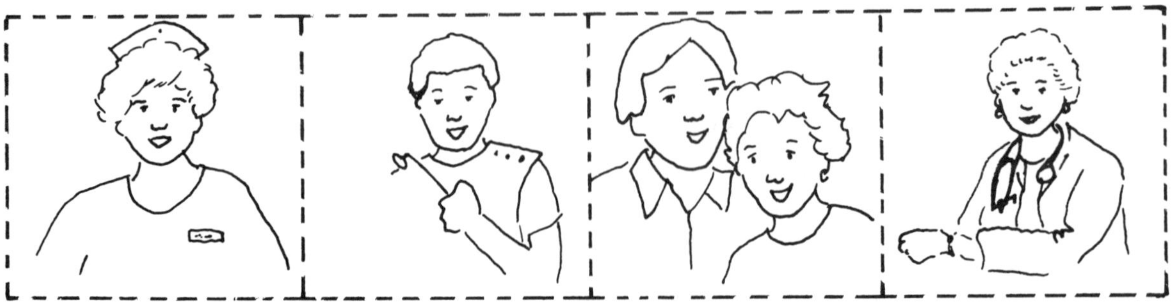

Name ______________________ Date ______________

TAKE CARE OF YOUR HEALTH *3–15D*

Here are some ways Susan takes care of her health. Write the number 1, 2, 3, or 4 in each box to show what Susan does first, second, third, and fourth each morning.

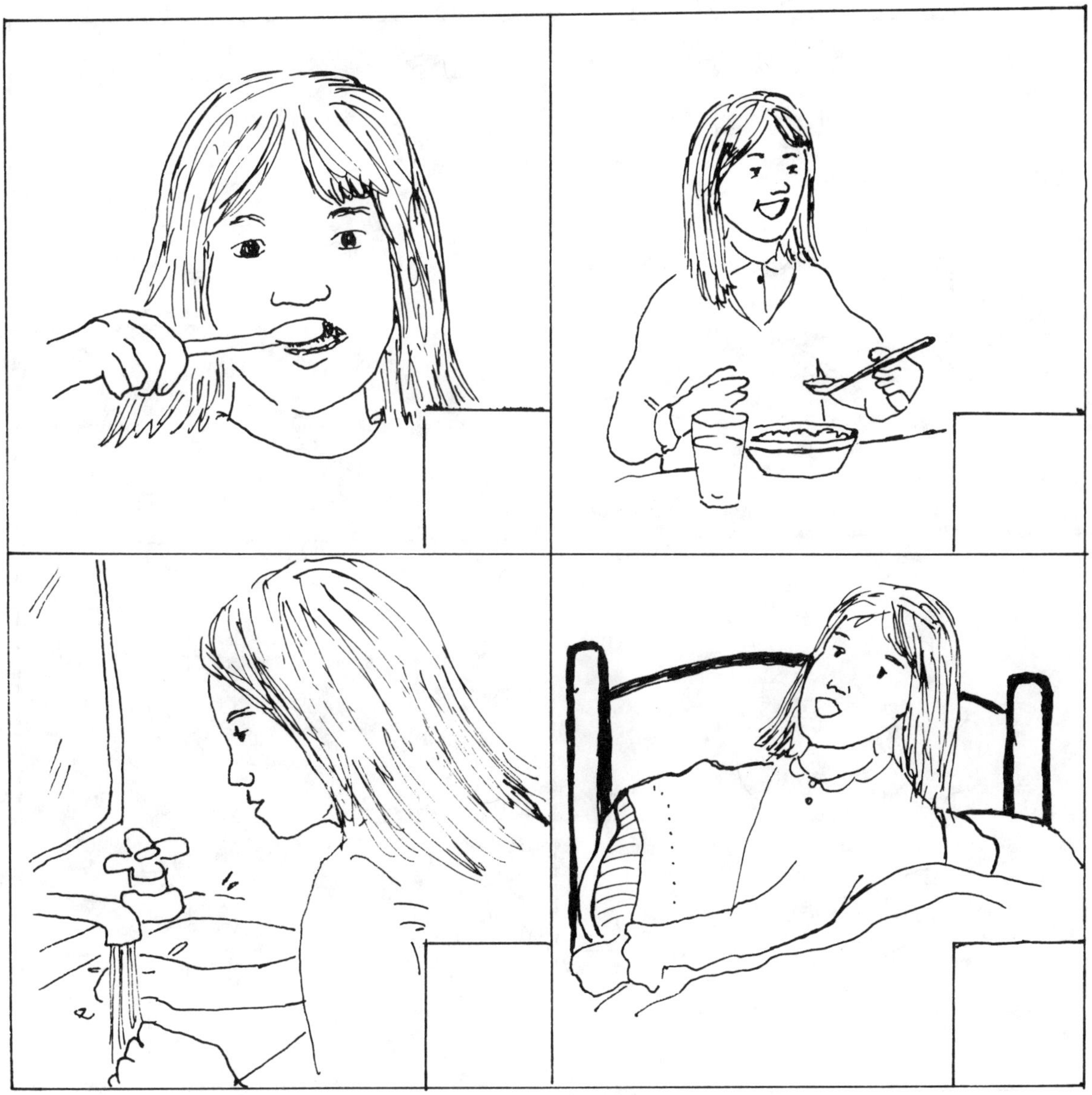

Name ________________________________ Date ________________

TAKE CARE OF YOUR HEALTH *3–15E*

Here are some ways Robby takes care of his health. Write the number 1, 2, 3, or 4 in each box to show what Robby does first, second, third, and fourth each day at lunch time.

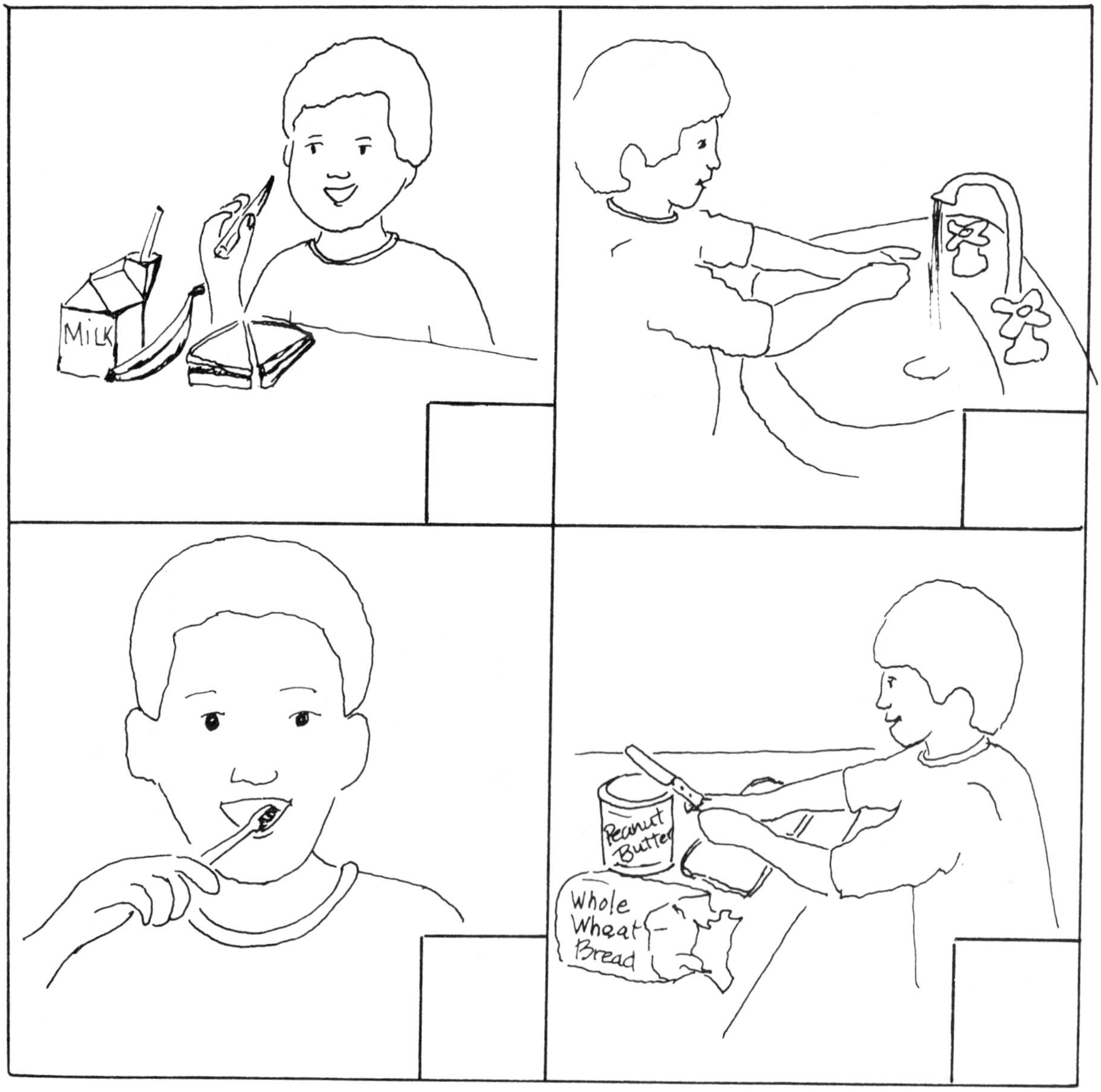

Name ____________________ Date ____________

GOOD GROOMING *3–15F*

In the picture story below, each picture stands for a word. Read the story and say the words for the pictures to find out the health message.

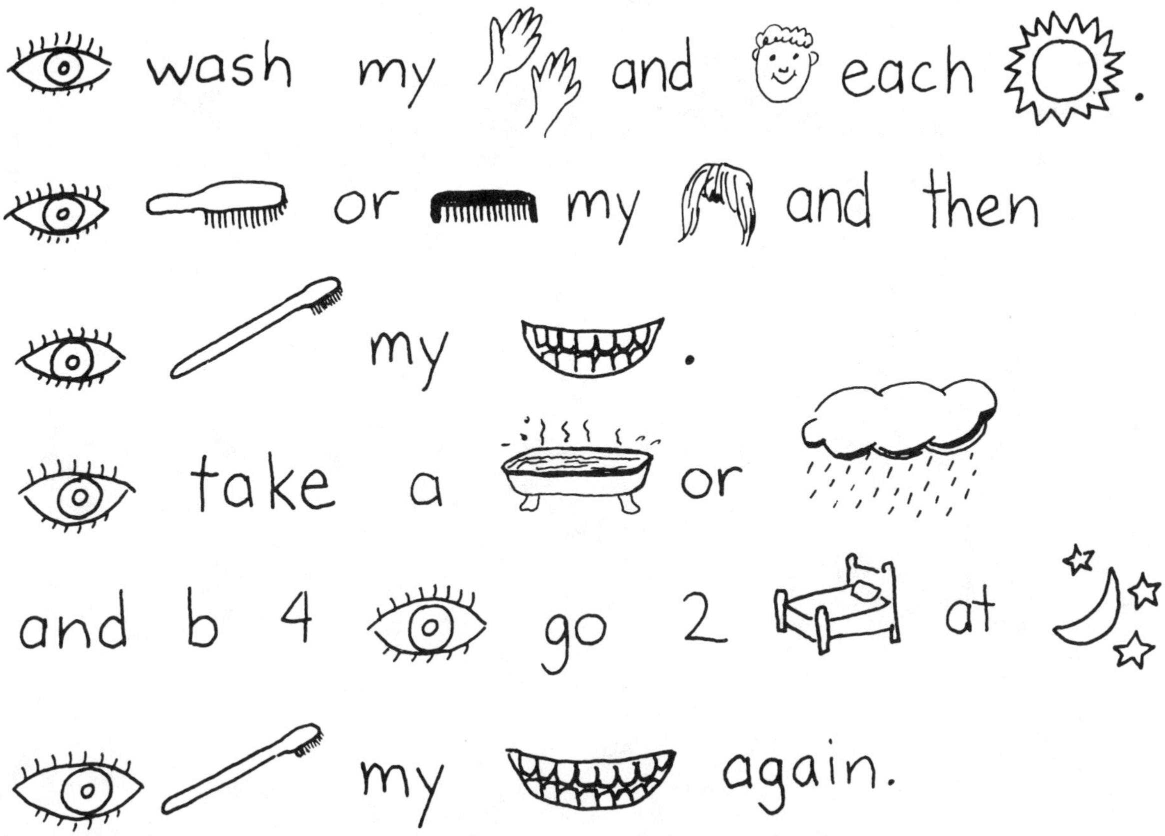

4 — FEELINGS AND SELF-ESTEEM

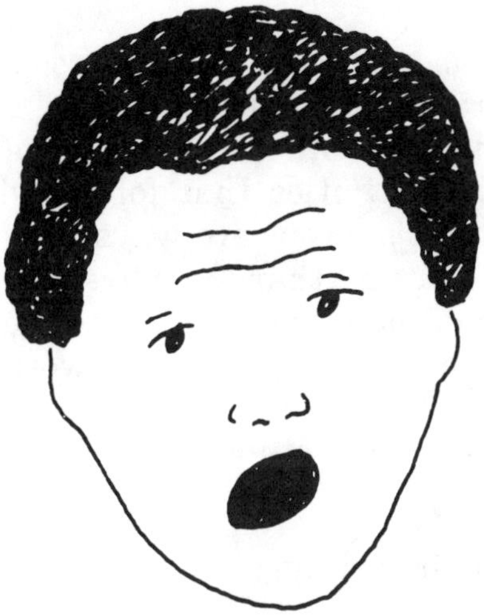

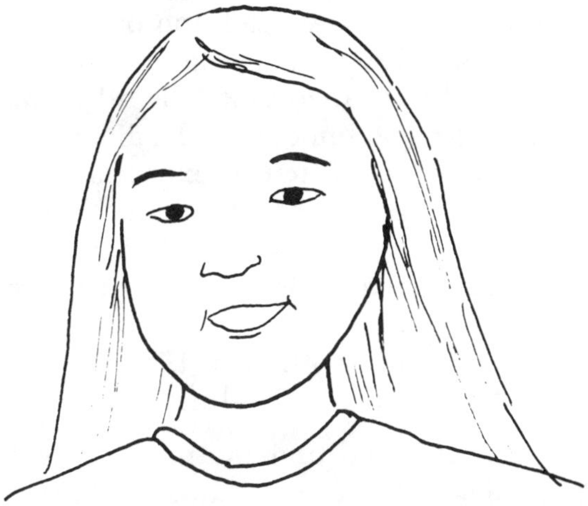

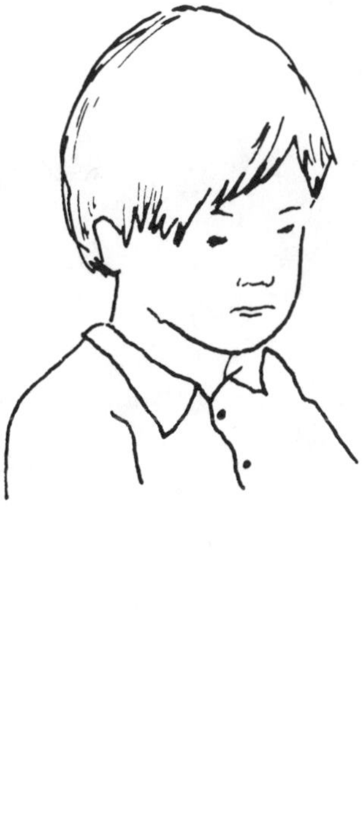

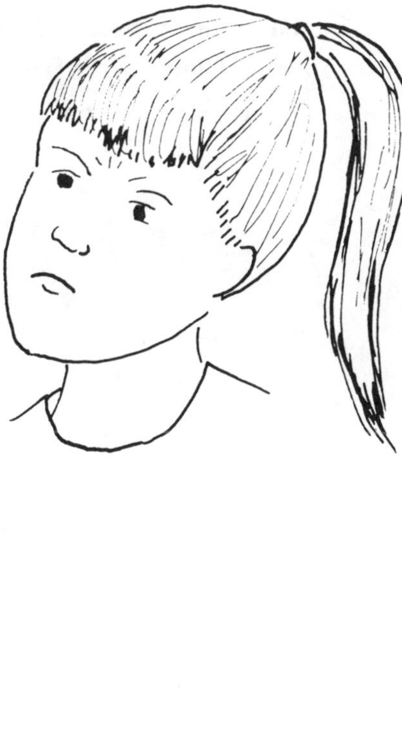

Self-esteem is a crucial factor in good health. Self-esteem is the way people feel about themselves; it affects their relationships with others and how they use the abilities that they have. People who do not like themselves have difficulty liking and getting along with others. In addition, students with low self-esteem often do poorly in school. By helping your students feel good about themselves, you can help them function more effectively in all areas of their lives.

Experts agree that self-esteem is a factor in substance abuse. Children who have low self-esteem are more likely to turn to alcohol or other drugs as a solution to their problems. Building students' self-esteem and helping them become more aware of their feelings will equip them to resist pressure to try alcohol and other drugs.

The ability to recognize, understand, and express feelings also contributes to good health. Children need to realize that it is all right to feel a wide range of emotions—anger, sadness, happiness, fear, excitement, pride, disappointment, frustration, and others. Children, as well as adults, often have difficulty expressing their feelings. The activities that follow will help students recognize their feelings and learn to express them in appropriate ways.

The activities in this section focus on mental health rather than on physical health. However, many health professionals believe that the health of the mind is linked to the health of the body. As students develop a better understanding of their feelings and self-worth, their overall health will be enhanced.

The activities in the Feelings and Self-Esteem section will help students:

- recognize and understand their feelings and emotions;
- develop and practice appropriate ways to express their feelings;
- recognize their own unique qualities and abilities;
- develop positive feelings of individuality, self-worth, and self-esteem;
- understand how their words and actions affect the feelings of others;
- learn effective techniques for getting along with others.

4–1 A PUPPET PAL

Learning to express feelings is important. A puppet pal can help students show and share their feelings.

Materials:

copies of Puppet Pal pattern 4–1A
brown paper lunch bags
crayons
scissors
glue
small bell

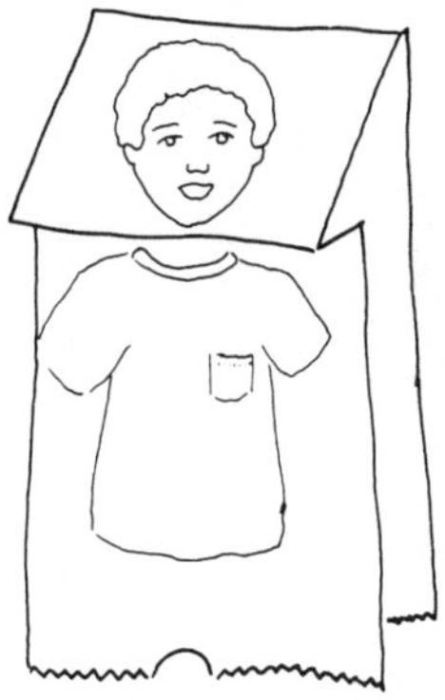

Directions:

Distribute the Puppet Pal patterns and have students color and cut out the head and body. Demonstrate how to glue the head of the puppet to the rectangular bottom portion of the lunch bag, and the body below. (See illustration.) Caution students not to glue the flap of the bag down.

When the puppets are finished, show students how to put one hand inside the bag, curl your fingers over the flap, and make the puppet "talk" by moving your fingers up and down. Then read the poem aloud.

Hello, puppet pal.
I'd like to hear
How are you feeling
While I am near?

Do you feel grouchy?
Do you feel sad?
Do you feel happy?
Do you feel mad?

Help the students learn the poem. Tell them to say it quietly to their puppets. Encourage them to have a conversation with their puppets about how they are feeling.

After a few minutes, ring the bell. Tell the students to move around the room and introduce their puppets to another puppet pal. Have them say the poem again with their puppets, and then have the puppets tell each other how they are feeling. Ring the bell several times so that students will have an opportunity to talk with several other puppet pals. Encourage students to use the puppet pals at home with their families.

4–2 FINGER PUPPET FAMILIES

Acting out family situations can help children understand and deal with their feelings.

Materials:

copies of Finger Puppets page 4–2A
scissors
crayons
transparent tape
envelopes for storing puppets

Directions:

Distribute the Finger Puppets pages. Have each student color four puppets, and then cut on the solid lines around each puppet. Help students tape the tabs on each puppet together to make a circle that will slip over one finger.

Organize students into groups of three. Assign each group one of these situations to act out:

1. Billy built a castle with blocks. When it was almost done, Jill accidentally bumped it and knocked it down. Billy cried and Aunt Teresa was angry with both children.
2. Grandpa worked all morning planting flowers in the garden. Just as he finished, Joe chased Rachel through the flower bed and crushed some of the new plants.
3. Mother promised to take Amy and Jeffrey to the zoo on Saturday. On Friday night, Mother said she had to work on Saturday and wouldn't be able to go to the zoo after all.
4. Katie and Brian drew pictures to give to their friend, Mr. Webster. Katie looked at Brian's picture and laughed. "That horse looks dumb," Katie said.

Move around the room and help students in each group decide who will play each part and how to dramatize the situation they have been assigned. Encourage students to discuss how the family members might feel, how they might express their feelings, and ways to resolve the situations.

Have groups take turns using their finger puppets to act out their situations for the class. After each presentation, lead the class in a discussion of times when they have been involved in similar situations, and encourage students to describe their feelings. Afterwards, have students store their puppets in envelopes until it is time to go home.

Extend the activity by reproducing additional Finger Puppets pages. Ask students to color and cut out the puppets. Trim off the tabs and glue a small square of felt to the back of each figure. Then have pairs of students arrange the figures on a flannelboard and use them to create and act out other family situations.

4–3 ME-IN-THE-MIRROR

Help students act out everyday feelings. Distribute small mirrors or have students face a wall mirror. Read the poem aloud and encourage students to watch their faces in the mirror as they follow the directions in the poem.

Hello, hello,
Me-in-the-mirror.
I'm so happy
To see you are here.
So wrinkle your nose,
Stick out your chin,
Look lonely, afraid,
Then happy again.
Waggle your tongue.
Tickle your hair.
Puff out your cheeks.
Push out the air.

Hold your head high,
Proud to be you.
Make a mad look.
Act frustrated, too.
Smack your lips loudly.
Giggle and frown.
Raise your eyebrows,
Then put them down.
Click your teeth fast
Then smile and sigh.
Me-in-the-mirror,
Good-bye. Good-bye.

4–4 WHAT'S HAPPENING?

Help students write their own stories about feelings.

Materials:

old magazines
scissors
glue
copies of What's Happening? activity sheet 4–4A

Preparation:

1. Cut out magazine pictures of children with a variety of facial expressions (happy, sad, afraid, angry, embarrassed, proud, ashamed, surprised).
2. Trim each picture so it is no larger than 4″ x 6″.

Directions:

Display the magazine pictures. Lead the class in a discussion of the facial expressions shown in some of the pictures. Talk about how the children in the pictures may be feeling.

Have each student choose a picture and glue it in the box at the top of his or her What's Happening? activity sheet. Then have students write answers to the questions on the sheet. Have younger students dictate their answers to the questions.

4–5 HOW DO YOU FEEL?

This activity will increase students' awareness of their feelings and why they feel the way they do.

Materials:

copies of How Do You Feel? activity sheet 4–5A
crayons

Directions:

Discuss common situations that children encounter, such as going to a birthday party, losing a favorite toy, getting hurt, and others. Ask students to describe how they think they would feel in each situation.

Distribute the How Do You Feel? activity sheets. Ask students to think of a time when they have felt happy, sad, or afraid. Ask each student to draw the way his or her face might have looked. Have students complete the sentence below the faces they drew. Younger students may dictate the rest of their sentences.

Extend the activity by having students complete additional sheets about other feelings.

4–6 HAPPY FACE, SAD FACE

Use puppets to help students recognize and deal with their feelings.

Materials:

- 9″ paper plates
- 2″ x 8″ cardboard strips for handles
- stapler
- crayons or markers

Directions:

Discuss common situations that make students feel happy, angry, sad, or afraid. Reassure them that everyone has such feelings and it's all right to feel that way.

Have students make puppets by stapling a cardboard handle to the edge of a paper plate. Then ask them to draw a happy face on one side of the plate and a sad face on the other side. Ask students to hold their puppets by the handles and show the side that shows how they are feeling right now. Some students may wish to share why they are feeling that way. If others prefer not to explain their feelings, don't pressure them.

Read the poem aloud. Ask students to turn the puppet back and forth to show the feelings described in the poem.

Happy face or sad face
It's up to me to choose.
Am I feeling happy
Or do I have the blues?

Smiley face or frowny face
As fast as one, two, three
I show how I'm feeling now
For everyone to see.

4–7 THE HAPPY LINE

It's wonderful to feel good about something and to share the good feelings with others.

Materials:

long piece of string or yarn
crayons
spring-type clothespins
drawing paper

Preparation:

1. Stretch the string or yarn across one end of the room or between two chairs.
2. Clip two clothespins on the line for each student.

Directions:

Ask the students to draw pictures of something which makes them feel happy. Encourage them to use favorite colors.

When everyone has finished drawing, read the poem aloud. Say it again and have students say it with you. Then have them chant the poem as they take turns clipping their pictures to the line.

Here's a happy picture
I want to share with you.
Maybe when you see it
You'll feel happy, too.

Let the students take turns describing their pictures and telling why they feel happy. Have them discuss why the pictures others drew make them feel happy, too.

Tell students to share their pictures at home. Let them draw, say the poem, and add new happy pictures to the line each week.

4–8 HAPPY HAT PARADE

March along and sing a song in the Happy Hat Parade.

Materials:

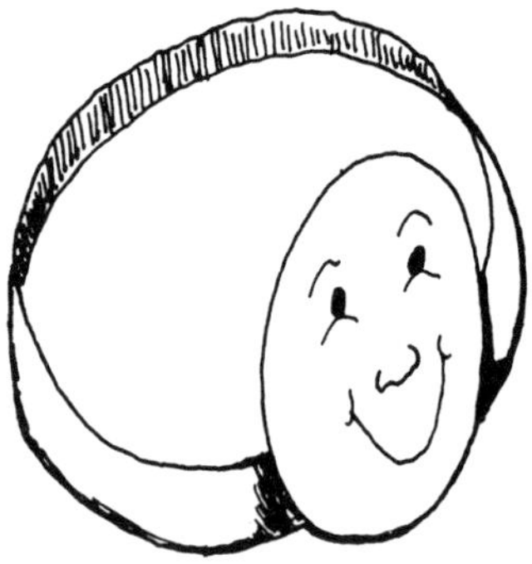

- white construction paper or lightweight cardboard
- ruler
- scissors
- stapler
- crayons

Preparation:

1. Cut 2″ x 24″ bands from construction paper or cardboard.
2. Cut a 6″ circle from construction paper for each student.
3. Staple a circle to the center of each band.

Directions:

Pass out the circles and bands. Have the students each draw a happy face on the circle, and decorate the band. Lap the ends of each student's band, forming a circle that fits his or her head, and staple the ends together.

Ask the students to put on their happy hats and form a line. Have them sing this song to the tune of "Mary Had a Little Lamb" as they march along:

Let's put on our happy hats,
Happy hats, happy hats.
Let's put on our happy hats
And march along the street.

Smiling in our happy hats,
Happy hats, happy hats.
Smiling in our happy hats
As we move our feet.

Marching in our happy hats,
Happy hats, happy hats.
Marching in our happy hats
We will prance along.

Happy in our happy hats,
Happy hats, happy hats.
Happy in our happy hats
With a happy song.

4–9 ANGRY FEELINGS

Help students understand that sometimes angry people say things that hurt others' feelings.

Preparation:

Print some of the following words on the chalkboard: stupid, dummy, weirdo, ugly, creep, nerd, four-eyes, know-it-all, fatso, skinny, sissy, wimp, shorty, klutz, baby, stuck-up, bonehead.

Directions:

Ask the students if they have ever been called any of the names on the board, and have them point to the names they were called. Discuss how they felt when they were called names. Then read the poem aloud.

When you feel angry
Wait and count to ten
Before you say something
That might hurt a friend.

One, two, three, four, five,
Six, seven, eight, nine, ten.
Throw away the angry words
And be yourself again.

Ask students to think about the poem. Then ask if they have ever been angry and called someone else a name. Have them tell how they felt being the name-caller. Discuss how an angry person may be sorry later about something he or she said and want to take the words back. Ask how counting to ten when they are angry might help.

Pair students with partners and have them practice how they might apologize to a person whom they have called a name. Discuss how saying "I'm sorry" to someone else makes them feel and how it makes the other person feel.

4–10 MAD BAG

Sometimes people feel angry with others or themselves. Help students make a punching bag to use when they are angry.

Materials:

pillowcase
heavy string or yarn
old newspapers

Preparation:

1. String a piece of yarn between two chairs.

Directions:

Have the students crumple several newspapers and stuff them into the pillowcase until it is three-fourths full. Twist the end of the pillowcase and tie it closed with a piece of string. Tie the pillowcase securely onto the line.

Explain to the students that it is all right to have angry feelings sometimes but that being angry does not give them an excuse to harm themselves or others.

Have the students line up and take turns punching the bag. Keep the "Mad Bag" hanging and encourage students to use it whenever they feel angry about something. Talk about other ways to ease anger: paint or color an angry picture, exercise, work with clay, talk about the anger, and other ideas.

Extend the activity by having each student make an individual "Mad Bag" from a paper grocery bag. Have students take their bags home to punch when they feel angry.

4–11 MUSICAL MOODS

Music makes people have many different feelings.

Materials:

record player or cassette player
records or cassettes (see suggestions)

Preparation:

1. Gather a selection of music which arouses different moods such as happy, sad, afraid, excited, or relaxed.
2. As an alternate activity, invite a musician to play music on an autoharp, flute, guitar, harmonica, piano, or recorder.

Directions:

Play the music for the students. Have them listen and move the way the music makes them feel. Ask them to sit down, close their eyes, and move to the music. Then discuss the feelings they had while listening to the music.

Suggestions for recordings or cassettes:

Peter and the Wolf, Leonard Bernstein, New York Philharmonic Orchestra, Columbia Records
Sorcerer's Apprentice, Fiedler, Leinsdorf, and Ozawa, Boston Symphony Orchestra, RCA Records
Grand Canyon Suite, Ferde Grofé, Alshire 101 Strings

4–12 UNIQUELY YOU

Help your students discover that each one of them is special and unique. Ask students to sit in a circle so they can see each other. Help them observe ways in which they are the same and different, such as height, hair color, eye color, and other characteristics. Then introduce the word *unique* and discuss its meaning: to be the only one of a kind; to be different from all others. Stress that although people may be the same in some ways, each one is unique and has his or her own personality, abilities, likes, and dislikes. Then use the following activities to help students recognize and understand ways in which they are unique.

I AM SPECIAL

Materials:

copies of I Am Special activity sheet 4–12A

Directions:

Distribute the I Am Special activity sheets. Lead students in a discussion of things they like and don't like. Have students write their likes and dislikes on their activity sheets, and then compare their lists.

ALL ABOUT ME

Materials:

- copies of All About Me activity sheet 4–12B
- ink pad
- basin of water, soap, towels
- crayons
- magnifying glasses
- small mirrors

Directions:

Distribute the All About Me activity sheets and the mirrors. Have students look in the mirrors to observe their hair and eye colors, and then fill in the blanks on their activity sheets.

Next, lead students in a discussion of things they like to do and do well. Help students recognize that there are many different areas in which they may excel such as sports, music, art, reading, writing, caring for people or animals, and others. Help them understand that each person is talented in at least one way. Then ask each student to draw a picture in the large box on the activity sheet of something he or she enjoys and does well.

To complete the activity sheet, help students discover that each one's fingerprints are different from those of anyone else. Help each of the students gently roll their fingertips across an ink pad, roll each inked fingertip across one of the five small boxes on the activity sheet, and then wash their hands. Distribute magnifying glasses and encourage students to compare fingerprints with one another. Have students add their completed activity sheets to their "Here's to My Health" booklet file folders.

WORDS ABOUT ME

Materials:

copies of Words About Me activity sheet 4–12C

Directions:

Distribute the Words About Me activity sheets. Talk with students about words that can be used to describe people such as helpful, happy, friendly, and others. Then help each child write four descriptive words about himself or herself in the numbered blanks on the activity sheet. Ask the students to write words that describe characteristics they like and don't like about themselves to complete the next two lines on the activity sheets.

Lead the students in a discussion of things they want to do or be when they are older. Include hobbies, sports, and other interests as well as occupations. Help the students complete the last two sentences on the activity sheets.

4–13 PRETTY PRINTS MURAL

Help students investigate more ways they are the same and different by making handprints and footprints.

Materials:

two 6′ lengths of butcher paper
newspapers
tempera paints in several colors
4 shallow trays
basin of water, soap, towels

Preparation:

1. Spread newspapers on the floor in an open area of the classroom.
2. Spread a 6′ length of butcher paper on top of the newspapers.
3. Pour a thin layer of paint into each of two shallow trays, and place the trays at one end of the butcher paper.
4. Place two chairs, the basin of water, the soap, and the towels at the other end of the paper.

Directions:

Ask students to remove their shoes and socks. Help them take turns gently stepping into the trays of paint with their bare feet, and then walking the length of the butcher paper. Hold each child's hand as he or she walks along to prevent slipping and falling. When the children reach the end of the paper, have them sit down to wash and dry their feet, and put on their shoes and socks. When the paint dries, write each child's name on one of his or her footprints.

Next, spread the other piece of butcher paper on a table and prepare two more trays of paint. Help the children take turns placing their palms in the paint, and then pressing them on the paper to make handprints. Provide a fresh basin of water and have the children thoroughly wash and dry their hands. When the paint dries, write each child's name on one of his or her handprints.

Display the footprint and handprint murals in the classroom. Encourage the children to compare sizes and other characteristics of the prints. Challenge them to find ways the handprints and footprints are the same and different.

4–14 STAR OF THE WEEK

Here's a way to help students get to know one another and learn what makes each one special.

Materials:

- Star of the Week pattern 4–14A
- My Home pattern 4–14B
- instant camera and film (optional)
- 3″ x 12″ cardboard strips
- glitter
- glue, brushes
- crayons
- drawing paper

Directions:

Set aside a section of the bulletin board for the "Star of the Week" activity. Copy the Star of the Week pattern, cut it out, and tack it at the top of the bulletin board section.

Choose a child each week to be the "Star of the Week." Take an instant photo of the child and tack it to the bulletin board below the star, or put up a picture the child has drawn of himself or herself.

Write the child's name in large letters on a cardboard strip. Have the child brush glue on the lines of the letters, and then sprinkle on glitter. Shake off the excess glitter and tack the name card to the bulletin board below the child's picture.

Fold 9″ x 12″ drawing paper in half and place the My Home pattern along the fold. Cut out the home and ask the child to color the front to resemble his or her home. Then have the child open the house shape and draw members of his or her family inside. If needed, help students write the names of family members.

Display the child's house along with his or her picture and name card. Let the child choose recent artwork and other materials to display also. During the course of the school year, make sure each student in the class has a turn to be the "Star of the Week."

4–15 SELF-ESTEEM BOOSTERS

Having good feelings about yourself is an important part of a healthy self image. Use these ideas in your classroom to boost your students' self-esteem.

WELCOME SONG

Sing this verse, to the tune of "Frère Jacques," as the children arrive or at the beginning of group activities. Encourage the other students to join in singing to one another.

Where is Eric? Where is Eric?
Here he is, here he is!
We are glad to see you,
We are glad to see you,
Yes, we are. Yes, we are.

Sing to several students each day. Keep track and be sure to include all the children each week.

HAPPY THOUGHTS

Materials:

plain envelopes
crayons
small slips of paper

Directions:

Have each student decorate the back of an envelope and write his or her name on it. Each day, tack two or three envelopes to the bulletin board, open side out. Pass out paper and ask the other students to write positive comments, one about each student whose envelope is on the bulletin board. When they finish, have students slip the papers into the envelopes. At the end of the day, the students may remove their envelopes from the bulletin board and take them home. Continue the activity until the envelopes of all the students in the class have been on the bulletin board.

GUESS WHO?

Help students recognize that they, and all people, have their own special qualities and talents. Ask students to each whisper to you something about themselves that makes them special and unique. Encourage them to describe personal qualities rather than material possessions or physical appearance. For example: "I'm friendly." "I'm a good reader."

Write what each student says on an index card. Shuffle the cards, and then read each one aloud. Ask students to guess who each statement describes. Give additional clues, as needed.

4–16 BLUE RIBBON WINNERS

Help students learn to appreciate their own and others' accomplishments.

Materials:

copies of Blue Ribbon pattern 4–16A, reproduced on blue paper, if possible
markers
masking tape

Preparation:

1. Cut out the Blue Ribbons.
2. Write a short phrase on each Blue Ribbon. Possible phrases: Spelling Champ; Terrific Thinker; Fantastic Friend; Hard Worker; Super Singer; Awesome Artist; and others.

Directions:

Keep a supply of Blue Ribbons on hand. Look for opportunities to present them to individual students, members of small groups, or the whole class.

Tell each of the students why they are receiving their Blue Ribbon. Then attach the ribbon to the student's clothing with a loop of masking tape rolled with the sticky side out.

A friendly pat, a hug, or a smile from you when you present the Blue Ribbons will help students realize that their efforts and accomplishments are important. Keep track and make sure each student receives a Blue Ribbon at least once a month.

4–17 QUIET SQUARE

Everyone needs time to relax and be quiet. A "quiet square" will provide a place to be alone even with others around.

Materials:

masking tape

Preparation:

1. Tape a 2′ x 2′ square on the floor for each student. Make sure the squares are a few feet apart.
2. Tape the children's initials in their squares.

Directions:

Ask the students if they enjoy being alone. Explain that the squares are spaces where they may spend some quiet time alone to sit and read, color, play a game, or just rest. Have a short quiet time each day.

Read the poem aloud. Help the students learn the poem and say it before each quiet time.

I zip my lips
And toss the key
To spend some time
Alone with me.

I like to rest
While I am there
In my special
Quiet square.

4–18 RELAXING RHYMES

Quiet time relaxes the body and relieves stress. Plan a quiet time for students at the same time each day.

Have the students sit comfortably a few feet apart. Ask them to shake their hands and feet, then take a deep breath and let it out. Tell them not to talk during quiet time. Softly read a relaxing rhyme and have the students act it out slowly.

Feather

Pretend you're a feather
Blowing in the breeze
Floating, floating, floating
High above the trees.
Floating, floating, floating
Slowly all around
Floating, floating, floating
Slowly to the ground.

Bubble

Blow up a giant bubble
And then climb inside.
Close your eyes. Get comfortable.
Take a magic ride.
Slowly you are rising
Toward the moon and stars.
Floating slowly upwards
Past Mercury and Mars.
Slowly you are turning
Up there in outer space
Then floating, slowly floating
Back to your starting place.

Cloud Bed

Spread out on a fluffy cloud
Arms and legs out wide.
Close your eyes and just relax
You're going on a ride.
Slowly, slowly, up you go
Floating overhead
Drifting with a gentle breeze
On a cloudy bed.
Then
Slowly, slowly down you float
Your cloud ride is through
So yawn and stretch and gently toss
Your cloud bed in the blue.

Activity Sheets for Section 4: Feelings and Self-Esteem

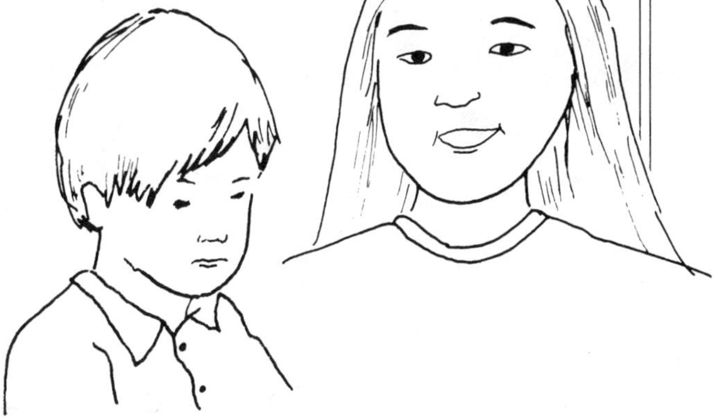

Name ________________________ Date ______________

PUPPET PAL

4-1A

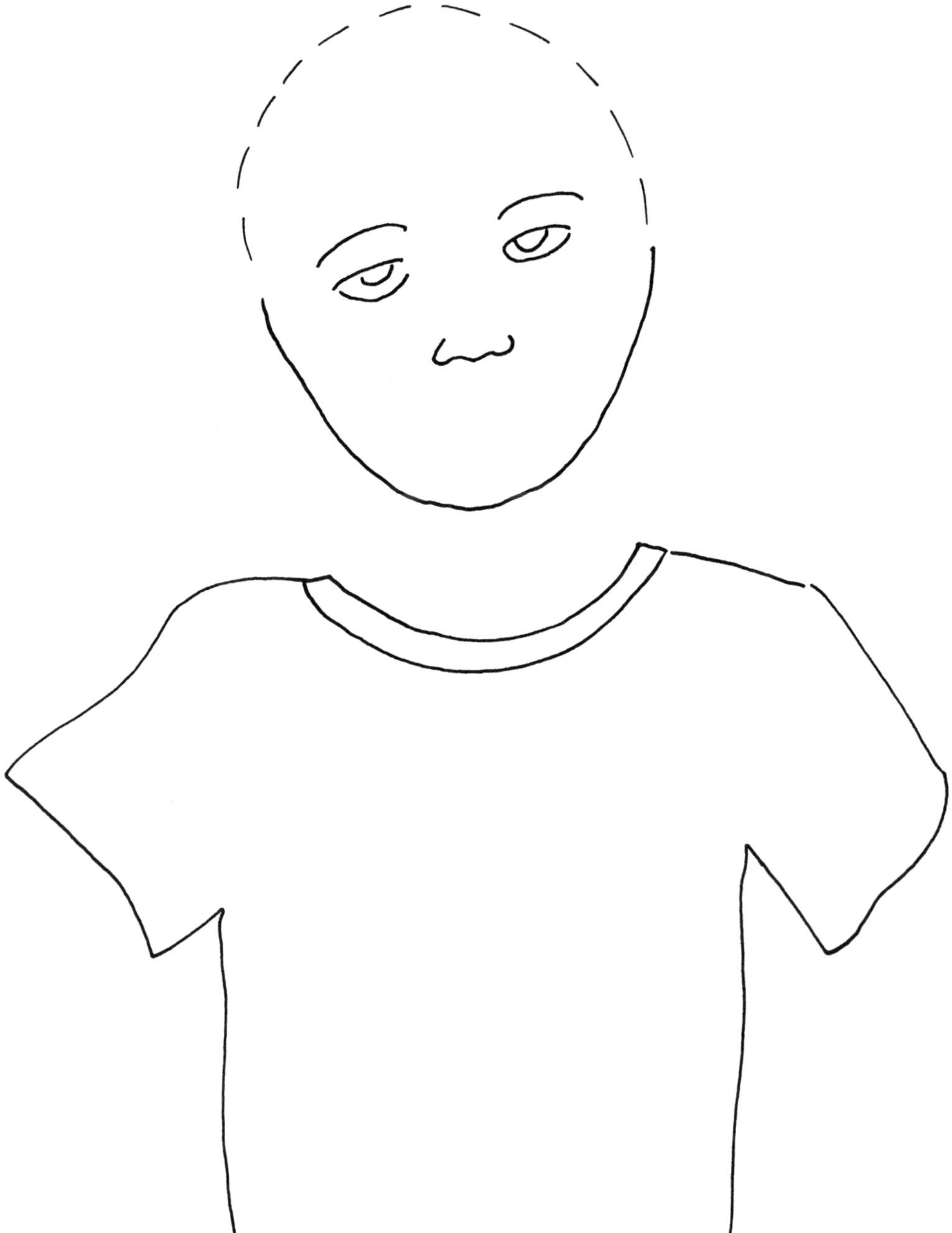

Name ______________________________ Date ______________

FINGER PUPPETS *4–2A*

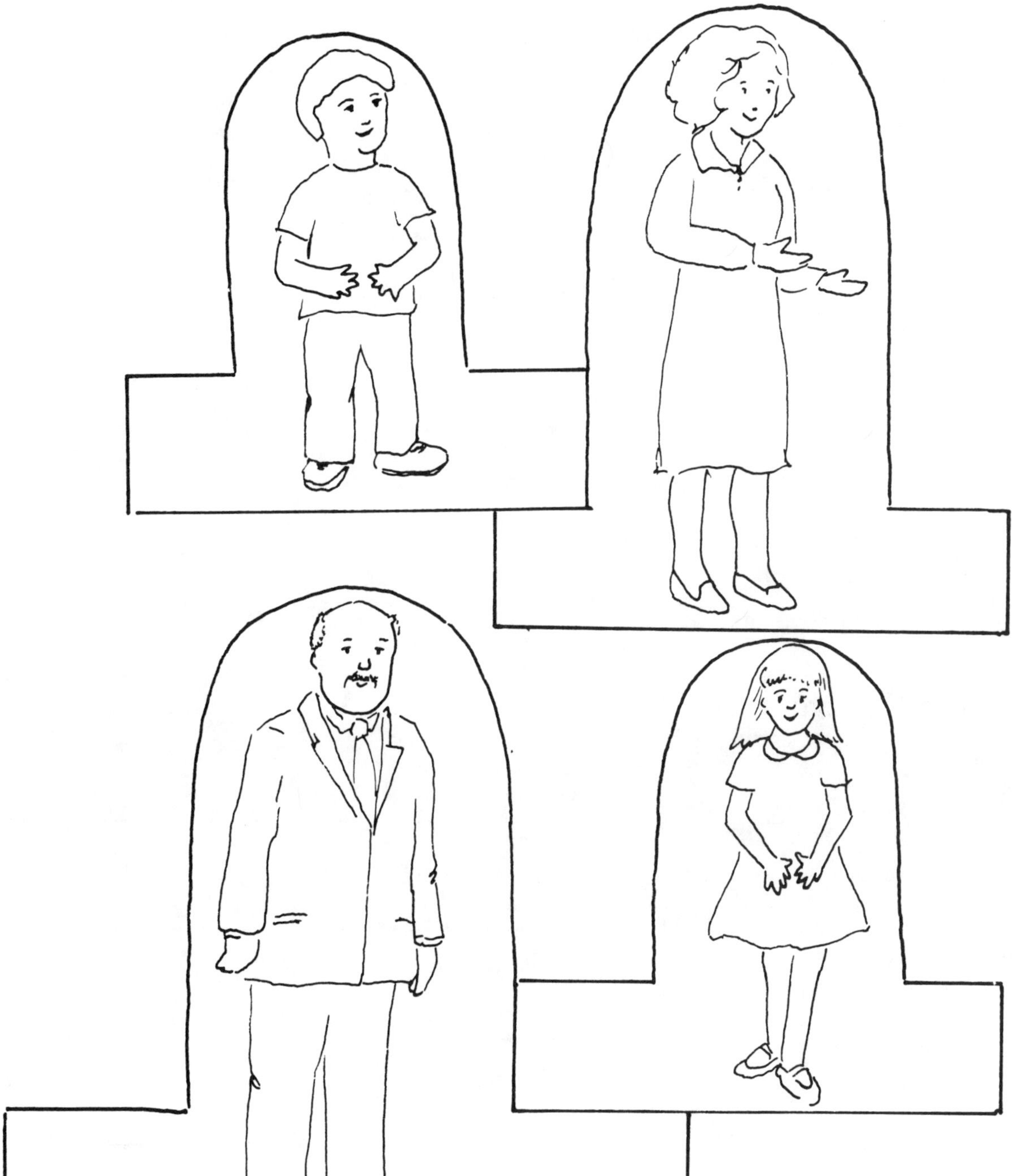

Name ______________________ Date ______________

WHAT'S HAPPENING *4–4A*

(glue picture here)

How does this child feel? ______________________

Why? ______________________

____

What will happen next? ______________________

____

____

Name ______________________________ Date ______________

HOW DO YOU FEEL? *4–5A*

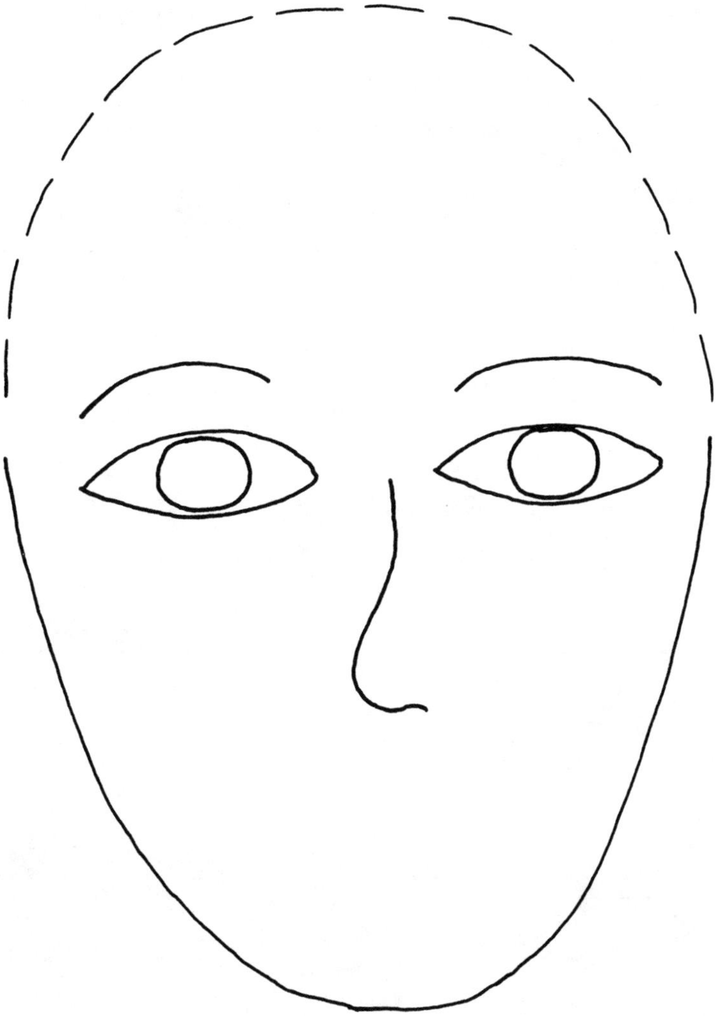

I feel ______________________ when ______________________

____

____.

Name ______________________ Date ______________

I AM SPECIAL *4–12A*

Things I Like | **Things I Don't Like**

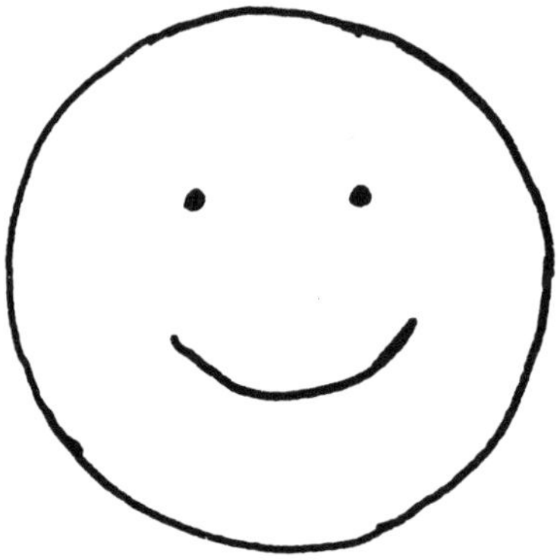

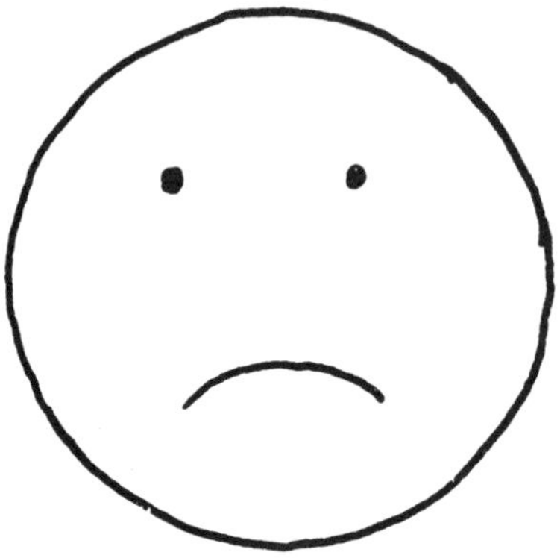

______________________ ______________________

______________________ ______________________

______________________ ______________________

______________________ ______________________

______________________ ______________________

______________________ ______________________

You are special. No one else is just like you. Write what you like and don't like. Then show your list to a friend. Did you write the same things?

Name ______________________________ Date ________________

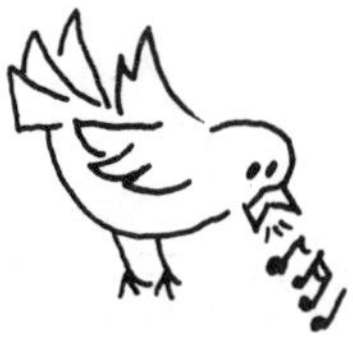

ALL ABOUT ME

4–12B

I have ______________________ eyes.

I have ______________________ hair.

This is what I'm good at.

My fingerprints

Name ______________________ Date ______________

WORDS ABOUT ME *4–12C*

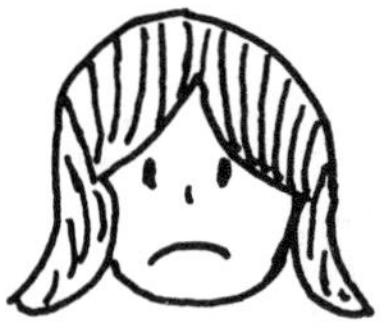

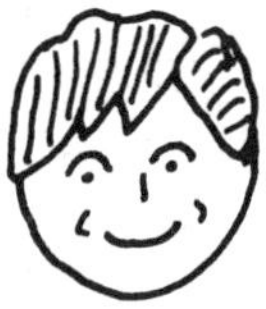

These words tell about me:

1. ______________ 2. ______________

3. ______________ 4. ______________

This is what I like about me:

____

This is what I don't like about me:

____

When I am 10 years old, I want to be:

____

When I am 20 years old, I want to be:

____

Name ______________________ Date ____________

STAR OF THE WEEK *4–14A*

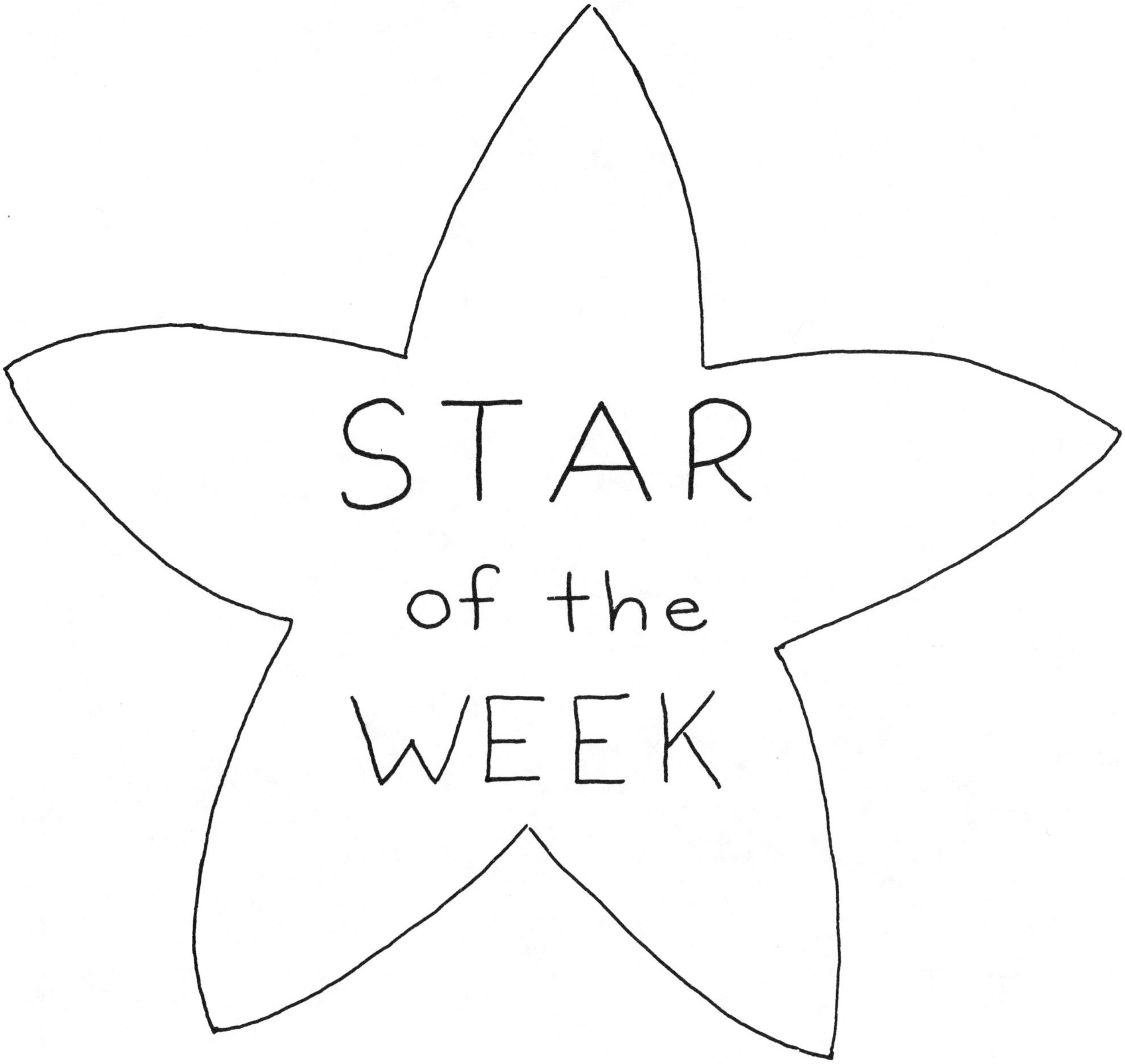

Name ______________________ Date ______________

MY HOME

4–14B

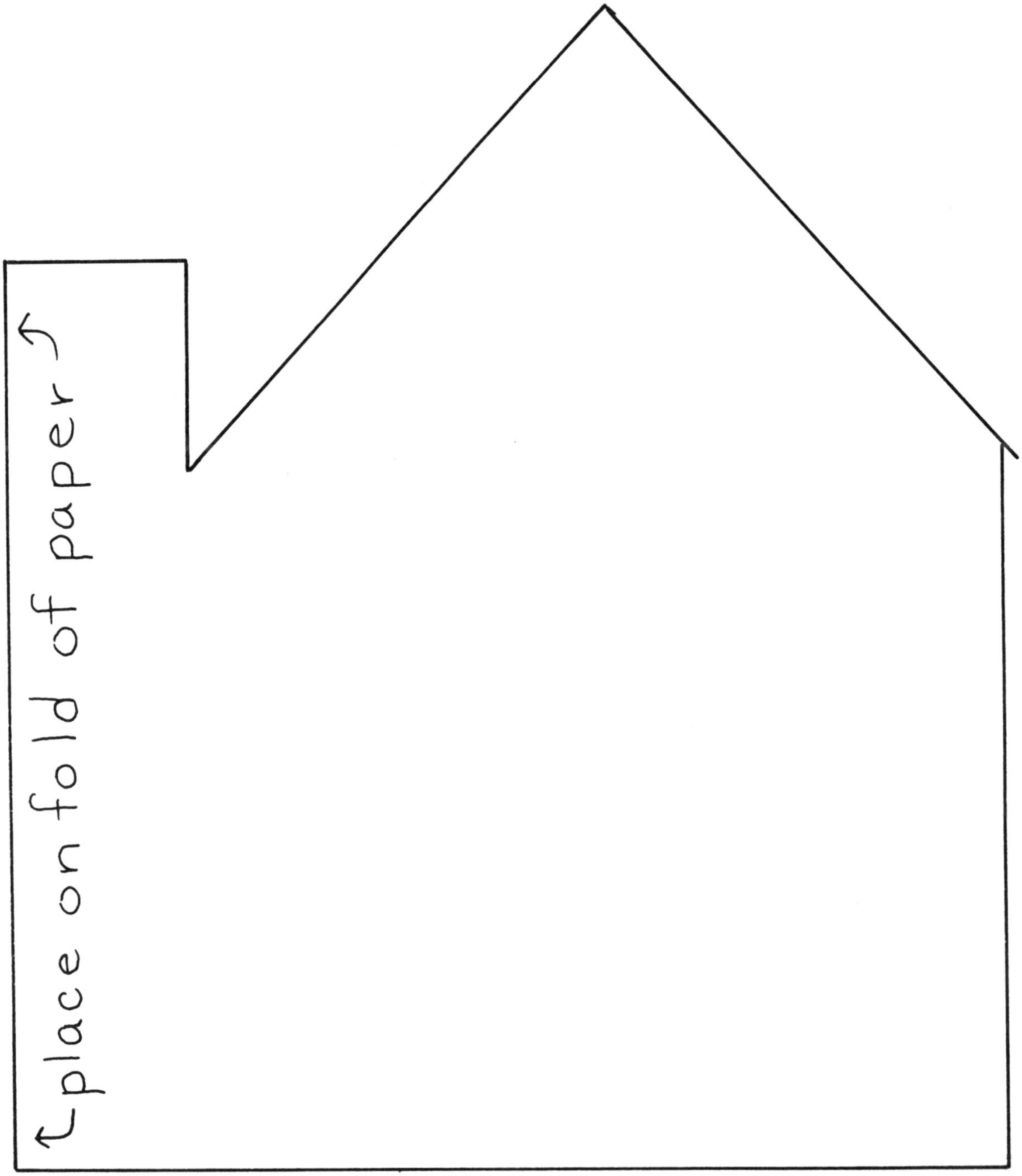

Name ______________________ Date ______________

BLUE RIBBON

4–16A

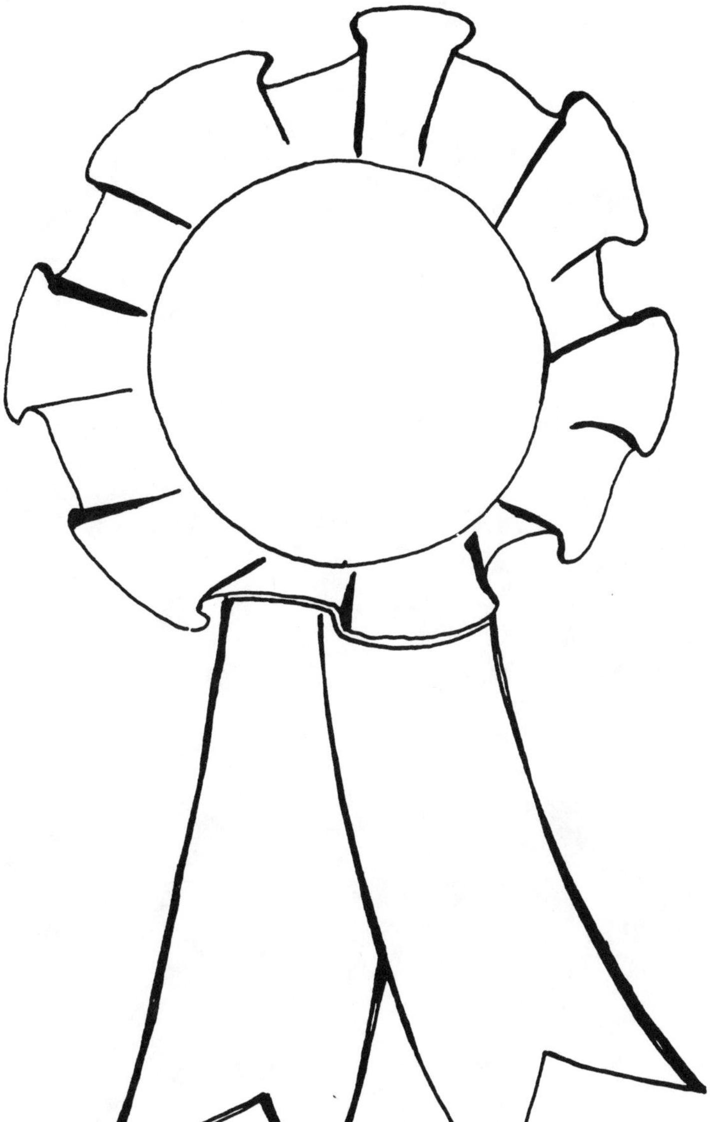

5 = SAFETY

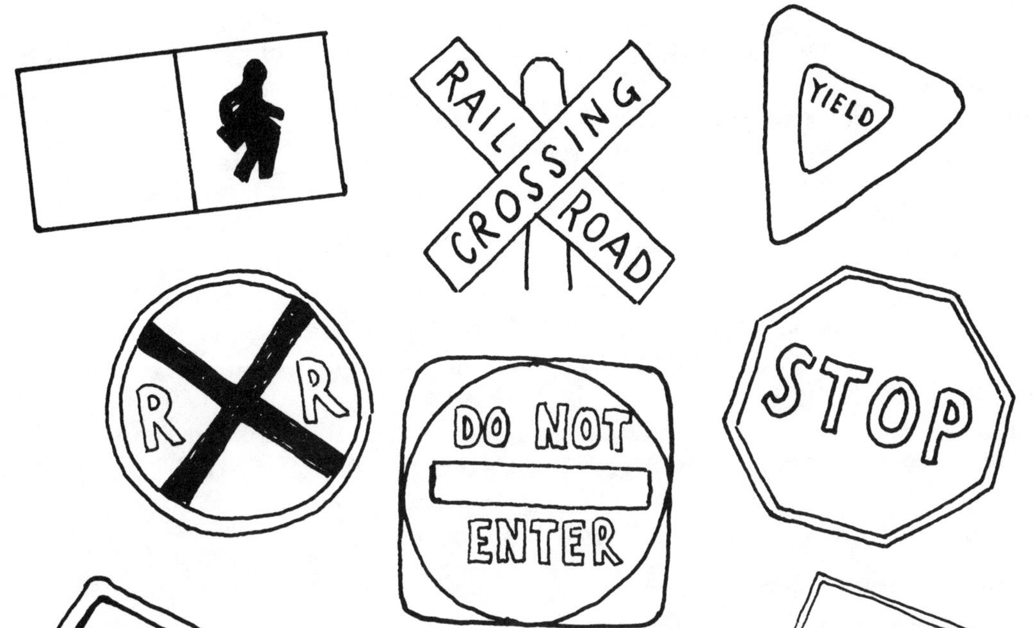
RAIL ROAD
CROSSING
YIELD
R R
DO NOT
ENTER
STOP
BIKE ROUTE
ONE WAY

Learning and practicing safety rules is an important part of staying healthy. Young children encounter many situations every day in which they must make decisions about the safe way to react. By introducing a variety of safety topics and helping students understand the safe responses to common situations, you can enable them to protect their own health.

The following safety topics are covered in this section: safety signs and symbols; how to respond to strangers; bicycle safety; kite safety; fire safety; safety in the home; how to call for help in an emergency. As you present the activities on each topic, make sure that the children understand the meaning of all the words that are used and that they know the right course of action to take.

Check your classroom carefully for hazardous materials and unsafe equipment or situations. Because children weigh less and have a higher metabolic rate, they are at greater risk than adults if they are exposed to hazardous materials. Check to be sure your art area is adequately ventilated, and have students wash their hands thoroughly after using art materials. Avoid using oil-based products, products containing solvents, powders or glitter that can be inhaled, and aerosol sprays.

Because role playing and game playing are effective tools for helping children learn and remember safety rules, this section contains suggestions for those activities. In addition, there are safety stories for students to read, a puzzle to cut apart and reassemble, and activity sheets for students to complete. You may wish to make additional copies of the games and the puzzle for students to use during free time.

Several review sheets are included which reinforce safety concepts presented in earlier activities. These sheets may be used for review, as independent activities, or they may be placed in learning centers.

The activities in the Safety section will help students:

- learn common safety rules;
- practice safe ways to participate in everyday activities;
- recognize objects and materials that are dangerous to their health;
- learn how to respond safely in situations they are likely to encounter at home, at school, or in their neighborhoods;
- learn how to react and how to call for help in an emergency.

5–1 READ THE SIGNS

Help students learn the meaning of common safety signs.

Materials:

copies of Safety Signs page 5–1A
crayons
scissors
glue
index cards or 3″ construction paper squares
record or cassette player
record or cassette of marching music

Preparation:

1. Cut one set of Safety Signs apart to make twelve individual signs.
2. Glue each sign to an index card or a construction paper square.

Directions:

Distribute the Safety Signs pages. Help students make sign cards, following the directions in "Preparation."

Have students spread their sign cards face up on their desks. Hold up your signs, one by one, and explain the meanings below. Ask students to find the matching signs on their desks.

Stop	Do not go any further. Make sure no cars are coming before you go.
Pedestrian Crossing	Make sure no cars are coming, then cross the street here. If you are riding a bicycle, stop for people in the crosswalk.
Don't Walk	The red hand below a traffic signal means "Don't Walk." Do not cross the street.
Walk	The figure of a person below a traffic signal means "Walk." You may cross the street but watch out for turning cars.
Bike Route	This is a safe place to ride your bicycle but watch out for traffic and parked cars.
School Zone	Make sure no cars are coming, then cross the street here. If you are riding a bicycle, stop for people in the crosswalk.

Railroad Crossing	You are coming near railroad tracks. Always stop, look and listen for trains.
One Way	Ride only in the direction the arrow shows.
Do Not Enter	Do not walk, ride, or go this way.
Yield	Let all the traffic pass before you enter or cross the street.
No Bicycles	Do not ride your bicycle here.

After explaining the meanings of all twelve signs, call on student volunteers to hold up signs and explain their meanings again. Then have students use their sign cards for the following activities.

SIGN CIRCLE

Lay two sets of cards face up on the floor in the shape of a circle. Play a marching song on the record or cassette player. Have students march around the outside of the circle. After a few moments, stop the music. Tell students to pick up the closest card and explain the meaning of the sign. Start the music again and repeat.

SIGN-UPS

Shuffle two or three sets of sign cards together. Hold up the signs, one by one. The first student to correctly identify each sign and explain its meaning keeps the card. When all the cards have been distributed, have students count to see who has the most.

SILENT SIGNS

Have students each spread their sign cards face up on their desks. Tell them that you will read the meaning of a sign. Ask them to hold up the sign that matches the meaning you have read. Continue until you have read the meanings for all 12 signs.

5–2 SAFETY SIGNS AND SYMBOLS

It is important for children to know what traffic signs and symbols mean.

Materials:

copies of Safety Signs page 5–1A
scissors
glue
craft sticks
crayons

Preparation:

1. Color a set of Safety Signs. Check in your neighborhood to see the proper sign colors.
2. Cut the signs apart.
3. Glue a safety sign to the end of a craft stick. Turn the stick over and glue another sign to the stick, back to back with the first sign.
4. Glue all the signs to craft sticks, making six double-sided safety signs.

Directions:

Pass out copies of the Safety Sign page. Show your colored signs, one by one, and ask students to locate the matching signs on their pages. Explain what each sign means as you hold it up. (See activity 5–1.) Ask students to repeat the sign names and meanings.

Help each student make six safety signs according to the directions in "Preparation." Have them glue the Walk and Don't Walk signs back to back on the same stick.

Read the safety poems aloud. Have students hold up the sign that matches each poem. Ask them to say the name of each sign aloud as they hold it up, and then tell what the sign means. Have students take their signs home and explain their meanings to their families.

Don't ride your bicycle
Where I'm on display.
Pick somewhere else
To pedal away.

I'm red and white
And you can tell
STOP. STOP. STOP . . .
Is what I spell.

Stop. Wait. Don't cross the street
When this hand is showing.
Wait until the Walk sign shows
Then you can start going.

When you get to school,
Cross the street right here.
Walk between the lines
When the traffic's clear.

Remember when you see me
Cross the tracks with care.
A train may be coming
While you are crossing there.

Ride your bike here.
This route is safe for you.
Ride here with your friends.
That's what you should do.

Bike one way only.
The arrow shows you where.
Bike one way only
When this sign is there.

Cross the street
Where you find
The pedestrian
Crossing sign.

5–3 HIDDEN SIGNS

Reinforce what your students have learned about common safety signs and symbols.

Materials:

copies of Hidden Signs activity sheet 5–3A
crayons

Directions:

Review with students the meanings of common safety signs and symbols (see activity 5–1). Then distribute crayons and the Hidden Signs activity sheets. Read the following directions aloud. After each one, give students time to find and color the sign described.

- Find the sign that shows where to ride your bicycle. Color the sign green.
- Find the sign that tells you to stop. Color the sign red.
- Find two signs that tell you to stop, look, and listen for trains. Color the round sign yellow. Draw a circle around the other sign.
- Find the sign that tells you which way to ride on a one-way street. Color the arrow white.
- Find the sign that tells you not to cross the street. Color the hand red.
- Find two signs that show where to cross the street safely. Color the signs yellow.
- Find the sign that shows that you may cross the street now. Draw a circle around the sign.
- Find the sign that tells you not to walk or ride this way. Color the space inside the circle red but leave the bar white.
- Find the sign that tells you to let all the traffic go by before you enter the street. Color the sign yellow.

5–4 SPIN-A-SIGN

Help students review the meaning of traffic signs they may see as they ride their bikes or go to and from school.

Materials:

copies of Spin-A-Sign page 5–4A
scissors
9″ paper plates
glue
pencils
paper fasteners

Preparation:

1. Cut out the Spin-A-Sign circle and the arrow from one Spin-A-Sign page.
2. Glue the Spin-A-Sign circle to a paper plate.
3. Line up the black dots on the arrow and the circle. Push a pencil point through both dots to make an opening. Attach the arrow to the circle with a paper fastener.

Directions:

Distribute a Spin-A-Sign page, a paper plate, and a paper fastener to each student. Show the Spin-A-Sign you have prepared, then help students assemble their own Spin-A-Signs, following the directions in "Preparation." When all the Spin-A-Signs are ready, have each student find a partner.

Tell one student in each pair to move the arrow on his or her Spin-A-Sign to point to one of the signs. Then have that student describe to his or her partner what that sign means without naming the sign. For example, for the Don't Walk sign the student might say, "This sign tells you that it is not safe to cross the street now." Tell the students to continue to give clues until their partners guess the sign and move their own Spin-A-Sign arrows to point to the same sign. Have partners take turns describing and guessing the signs until they have covered all 12 signs pictured.

5–5 WATCH THE SIGNAL

Help the students learn the meanings of the lights on a traffic signal.

Materials:

copies of Traffic Signal activity sheet 5–5A
6″ construction paper circles (1 red, 1 yellow, 1 green)
red, yellow, and green crayons

Directions:

Hold up the red paper circle and ask students to identify the color. Explain that a red light on a traffic signal means they should stop and not cross the street. Repeat with the yellow and green circles, explaining that a yellow light means that the signal is about to change to red, and that a green light means they may cross the street but they should still watch out for cars.

Play a game with students to reinforce the meanings of the traffic signal lights. Have students line up side by side about 20 feet away, facing you. Give these movement directions:

Green:	Walk slowly toward the leader.
Yellow:	Walk in place but do not move forward.
Red:	Stop walking and wait for a green light.

Randomly hold up the construction paper circles, one at a time. Show each circle for a few seconds, and then show a different circle. When students are familiar with the game, let them take turns being the leader.

Read the following poem aloud, and then have students repeat it with you.

Watch the signal
Up near the top.
Red, red, red light
Means stop, stop, stop.

Watch the signal,
Yellow's in it.
Yellow light means
Wait a minute.

Watch the signal
So you will know.
Green, green, green light
Means go, go, go.

Distribute the Traffic Signal activity sheets. Help students read the directions and complete the sheet.

5–6 EXIT SIGN

Knowing what the word *EXIT* means is important in an emergency.

Materials:

copies of Exit Sign activity sheet 5–6A
red construction paper
glue

Directions:

Show a copy of the Exit Sign activity sheet and read the word EXIT aloud with students. Spell the word aloud and have students repeat each letter after you.

Explain that exit signs show where the doors are in a building. Discuss times when people might need to leave a building quickly such as in a fire, an earthquake, or other emergencies. Take students on a walk around the school to look for EXIT signs.

In the classroom, emphasize that even in an emergency, it is important not to run or push to get out of the building. Have students practice walking carefully but quickly to the nearest exit.

Pass out copies of the Exit Sign activity sheet. Help students read the directions and complete the sheet.

5–7 POISON PUZZLE

It is important for all children to recognize the poison symbol and know its meaning.

Materials:

copies of Poison Puzzle page 5–7A
black crayons
scissors
envelopes for storing puzzle pieces

Directions:

Show a copy of the Poison Puzzle and tell students that this is an important symbol to know and remember. Say the word *poison* and have students repeat it with you. Explain to students that the poison symbol is put on bottles or cans which contain things that could make them very sick. Emphasize that they should never touch anything labeled with the poison symbol.

Distribute copies of the Poison Puzzle. Have students color the skull and crossbones black but leave the teeth and background white. Then show how to make a puzzle by cutting the picture apart on the lines. Help students put the puzzle pieces together to make the poison symbol again.

Pass out envelopes in which students can store their Poison Puzzle pieces. Encourage them to ask their parents to check at home for containers marked with the poison symbol, and then place the containers on high shelves out of the reach of young children.

5–8 SAFETY STORIES

Help students practice the safe response to situations they may encounter.

Materials:

copies of Safety Stories 5–8A through 5–8D

Directions:

Distribute the Safety Stories and read each story aloud as students follow along. Discuss safe responses for each situation and help students act them out. Emphasize the following safety concepts:

- People are strangers unless you or your parents know them well and know their names and addresses.
- Never go anywhere with a stranger.
- Never take anything from a stranger.
- If a stranger asks you questions, don't answer.
- If a stranger asks you to get in a car, shout NO! Run away and find an adult you know.
- Don't believe a stranger who says your parents sent him or her to get you. Run away and find an adult you know.
- Don't open the door when you are home alone.
- Always walk to and from school and other places with a friend.

Have students complete the Safety Stories by writing what the children in each situation should say or do. Younger students may dictate their responses.

Safe responses:

Story 1–Sean should tell the caller his mother cannot come to the phone but he will take a message for her.

Story 2–Emily should leave the door closed and ask the person to leave the package on the doorstep.

Story 3–Megan and Jacob should not get into the car. They should shout NO! and run away, then find an adult they know.

Story 4–Jessica should not walk home alone. She should either wait for her friends or call home and ask someone to come and get her.

5–9 BICYCLE SAFETY

Children need to learn how, when, and where to ride their bicycles safely.

Materials:

copies of Bicycle Safety activity sheet 5–9A

Directions:

Discuss with students the following DO's and DON'T's for safe bicycle riding.

DO

- Wear a helmet.
- Obey traffic rules and signs.
- Wear shoes that protect your feet.
- Ride in a safe place, away from heavy traffic.
- Watch out for cars, and for people who are walking.
- Watch out for cars backing out of driveways.

DON'T

- Wear sandals.
- Ride barefoot.
- Wear long scarves, baggy pants, or other clothing that might catch in the bicycle chain.
- Give a friend a ride on your bike.
- Ride after dark.

When students understand the DO's and DON'T's and the reasons for them, randomly read aloud several rules from each list. Have students give a "thumbs up" signal if the rule is something they should do, and "thumbs down" if it is something they should not do.

Distribute the Bicycle Safety activity sheets. Help students read the directions and complete the sheet.

5–10 KITE-FLYING FUN

Teach students how to "go fly a kite" safely.

Materials:

copies of Kite Pattern page 5–10A
scissors
crayons
hole puncher
gummed reinforcements
string
crepe paper streamers
stapler

Directions:

Ask students to tell about times when they may have flown kites. Have them tell where they flew their kites, what their kites looked like, and what kind of day it was.

Discuss the following kite safety rules with students:

- Kites should be made of string, wood, and paper.
- Never use metal, wire, metallic string, or metallic cloth.
- Always fly a kite in a large open area, away from the street, power lines, trees, and TV antennas.
- Never fly a kite in the rain or during a lightning or thunder storm.
- If your kite gets caught in power lines, ask your parents to have a firefighter or a power company worker get it down. NEVER try to get it down yourself.

Distribute the Kite Pattern pages. Have students color and cut out the kites. Help each student punch a hole at the top of the kite, strengthen the hole with gummed reinforcements, and tie a string through the hole. Give students crepe paper streamers to staple to their kites for tails.

Read aloud the sentence below and then read the phrases that follow, one at a time. Tell students to hold their kites high if the words describe a safe way to fly a kite. If not, students should keep their kites on their desks.

John and Sandy flew their kites:
at the football field
in the street
at the park
in the rain
in the woods
on a sunny day
by the power poles

Clear an open space in the classroom and have students spread out, holding their kites. Read the following poem aloud and have students do the motions.

Run with the wind and
Hold your kite high.
Make it go dancing
Across the sky.
Dipping and darting
Up by the sun,
Everyone's having
Kite flying fun.

5–11 WHAT'S SAFE? WHAT'S NOT?

Children can learn to handle some objects carefully; they should never touch other objects at all. Help your students learn the difference.

Materials:

copies of Do Not Touch/Handle With Care picture page 5–11A
scissors
index cards or 3″ construction paper squares
glue

Preparation:

1. Cut one set of Do Not Touch/Handle With Care pictures apart to make 12 individual pictures.
2. Glue each small picture to an index card or a construction paper square.

Directions:

Distribute the Do Not Touch/Handle With Care picture pages. Have students make picture cards, following the directions in "Preparation."

Work with a small group of students and have them spread their picture cards face up on their desks. Hold up your set of pictures, one by one. Ask students to identify each object and find the matching picture on their desks. Help students decide which objects they may handle carefully (knife, scissors, iron, matches, saw, hammer and nails) and which they should never touch (gun, poison, razor, ax, firecrackers, broken bottle).

Discuss the following safety rules for using the Handle With Care objects:

- Before using any of the objects, have your parents or another adult show you how to use it safely.
- Never run with sharp objects such as knives or scissors.
- Carry knives and scissors with their points down.
- Never play with matches.
- Always unplug an iron when you finish using it.

Ask students to find partners for the following games.

SORT THE PICTURES

Using two sets of picture cards, ask each pair of students to classify the objects, making one group of objects that may be handled carefully and another group of objects that should not be touched.

WHAT IS IT?

Have pairs of students shuffle one set of picture cards thoroughly and place them face down in a pile. Tell students to take turns drawing the top card and describing the object to their partners. For example: It is sharp and pointed. You can cut paper with it. What is it? (scissors) Tell students to continue to give clues until their partners correctly guess the name of the object. Then have partners decide together if the object can be handled carefully and why or why not.

MEMORY GAME

Ask pairs of students to shuffle two sets of picture cards thoroughly and then spread them out, picture side down, on a table. Tell students to take turns turning over two cards. If the pictures match, the student should identify the objects, tell whether they may be handled carefully or should not be touched, and then keep the cards. If the pictures do not match, they should be turned face down again. Students should continue to play until all the cards have been matched.

5–12 FIRE DRILL

Everyone must learn, remember, and practice fire safety rules.

Tell students it is important to know the way to get out of the building quickly and safely in case of fire. Have them practice a fire drill. Emphasize the following fire drill safety rules:

- Do not run! Get in line quickly with your classmates.
- Listen for instructions from the teacher or an adult in charge.
- Walk calmly and quickly outside to a central meeting place.
- Wait quietly in line with your class.
- Listen for the "all clear" bell.
- Wait and listen for directions from your teacher or an adult in charge.
- Walk safely back to the classroom when your teacher or an adult in charge tells you it is all right.

Read aloud the 911 poem in Safety Verse (activity 5–16) and ask the students to do as the poem tells them. Have them practice dialing 911 or their emergency number on a real telephone (unplugged) to report a pretend fire. Explain carefully that they are to dial the emergency number on another phone only in case of a real fire or another emergency. Stress that it is important to keep emergency phone lines open for reporting real emergencies.

5–13 STOP, DROP, AND ROLL!

It is important to teach students what to do in case their clothes catch fire.

Materials:

red felt
scissors

Preparation:

Use the flame pattern to cut a red felt flame for each student.

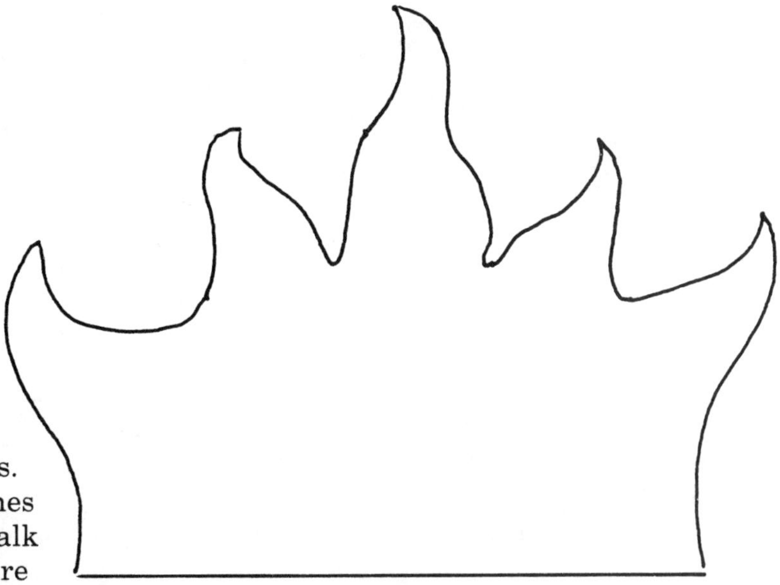

Directions:

Give each of the students a flame and tell them to put it on their clothes. Inform students that if their clothes catch fire they should not run or walk around because air will keep the fire going. Show them how to drop to the floor or ground and cover their faces with their hands. Tell them to keep rolling over slowly until the fire is out.

Read the following poem aloud and have the students do the motions:

STOP! STOP! STOP!
Drop to the ground.
Cover your face and
Roll slowly around.

Help students learn the poem, and then ask them to chant it several times. Encourage them to teach family members how to stop, drop, and roll.

5–14 HOME FIRE SAFETY

Encourage students and parents to plan a home fire drill.

Materials:

copies of Indoor and Outdoor Fire Safety activity sheets 5–14A and 5–14B
copies of Escape Route activity sheet 5–14C

Preparation:

Make arrangements for students to visit a fire station or invite a firefighter to visit the classroom.

Directions:

Introduce the firefighter to the students and ask him or her to talk about home fire safety. Ask the firefighter to show the students some fire fighting equipment and explain how it helps him or her fight fires. Let the students try on a face mask, fire helmet, air tank, and other equipment.

After the firefighter's visit, talk with students about planning a home fire drill. Emphasize the following home fire safety rules:

- Decide on two safe escape routes.
- Choose a central meeting place away from the house or apartment.
- Leave the building quickly.
- Cover your nose and mouth with a damp cloth to keep from breathing too much smoke.
- Never go back into a burning building.
- Wait at the central meeting place.

Read the following fire safety rules aloud and encourage students to discuss them with their parents. Suggest that parents and children work together to make sure their home is free from fire hazards.

- Put emergency numbers by the telephone.
- Check to see if smoke detectors are working.
- Never play with matches. Keep them away from younger brothers and sisters.
- Do not play near a stove or fireplace.
- Get rid of old newspapers and trash that could catch on fire.
- Keep a working flashlight in every room.
- Practice stop, drop, and roll with your family.

Distribute the Fire Safety activity sheets. Help students read the directions and complete the sheets. Send home an Escape Route activity sheet with each student.

5–15 CALLING FOR HELP

Knowing how to call for help can make a crucial difference in an emergency.

Materials:

copies of Emergency Number activity sheet 5–15A
red crayons
play telephones

Preparation:

Find out the telephone number to call for emergency services in your area.

Directions:

Write the emergency number on the chalkboard and have students chant it in unison several times. Explain that they should only dial this number when someone is badly hurt or needs help quickly.

Organize student pairs and give each pair a play telephone. Let one student play the part of the emergency operator while the other one pretends to report an emergency. Tell the callers to begin by saying, "This is an emergency." Then have them give their names and addresses and tell what the emergency is, who is involved, and when and where it happened. Stress that they should not hang up, but stay on the phone in case the operator needs to ask questions. Then have partners switch roles so both have turns to be the operator and the caller.

Distribute the Emergency Number activity sheets and red crayons. Help students read the directions and complete the sheet. Have students add their completed activity sheets to their "Here's to My Health" booklet file folders.

5–16 SAFETY VERSE

Good safety habits help protect everyone.

Read the safety verse aloud to the students and have them act out the motions.

When you have an emergency
Dial 911 (or your emergency number*) and say
Your name and address clearly
So help can come your way.
Dial 911. Dial 911.
That's what you have to do
For giving information
So help will come to you.

*If there is a different emergency number in your area, substitute it for 911.

Before you cross
Look all around
Then you can move your feet.
Before you cross
Look all ways
Then walk across the street.

Buckle up your seatbelt
When you get in a car.
Buckle up for short rides
Or if you're going far.
Buckle up your seatbelt
Tell everyone inside.
Buckle up for safety
And a happy ride.

Fingers in your lap
When someone shuts the door.
Buttons down. Buckle up.
Don't play anymore.
Talk or sing quietly
Or watch the things outside.
But don't disturb the driver
When you're off on a ride.

Have the students chant this safety poem:

Inside, outside, home, school, away.
Safety first is best each day.
Safety first by everyone
Makes for inside, outside fun.

5–17 SAFETY REVIEW SHEETS

This is a good time to review what the children have learned about safety.

Materials:

copies of review sheets 5–17A through 5–17C
pencils

Directions:

Have copies of these review sheets available. They may be used for review, as independent activities, or they may be placed in learning centers.

Activity Sheets for Section 5: Safety

5–1A	Safety Signs
5–3A	Hidden Signs
5–4A	Spin-A-Sign
5–5A	Traffic Signals
5–6A	Exit Sign
5–7A	Poison Puzzle
5–8A	Safety Story 1
5–8B	Safety Story 2
5–8C	Safety Story 3
5–8D	Safety Story 4
5–9A	Bicycle Safety
5–10A	Kite Pattern
5–11A	Do Not Touch/Handle With Care
5–14A	Indoor Fire Safety
5–14B	Outdoor Fire Safety
5–14C	Escape Route
5–15A	Emergency Number
5–17A	Safety Code
5–17B	Draw-A-Sign
5–17C	Safety Puzzle

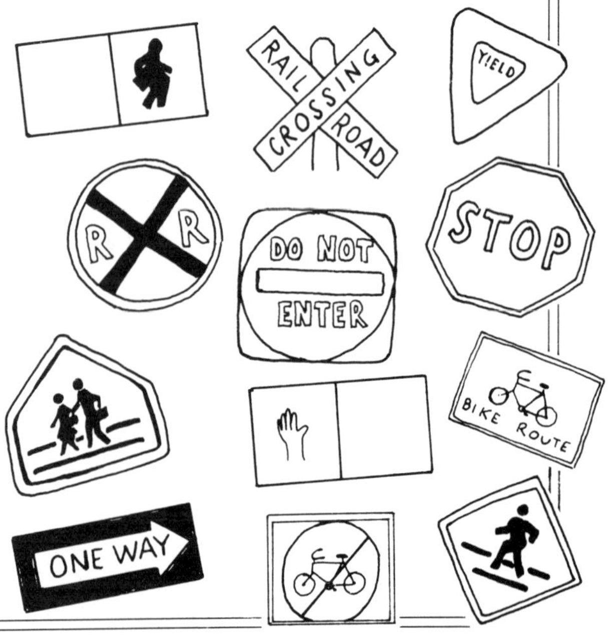

Name ______________________ Date ______________

SAFETY SIGNS *5–1A*

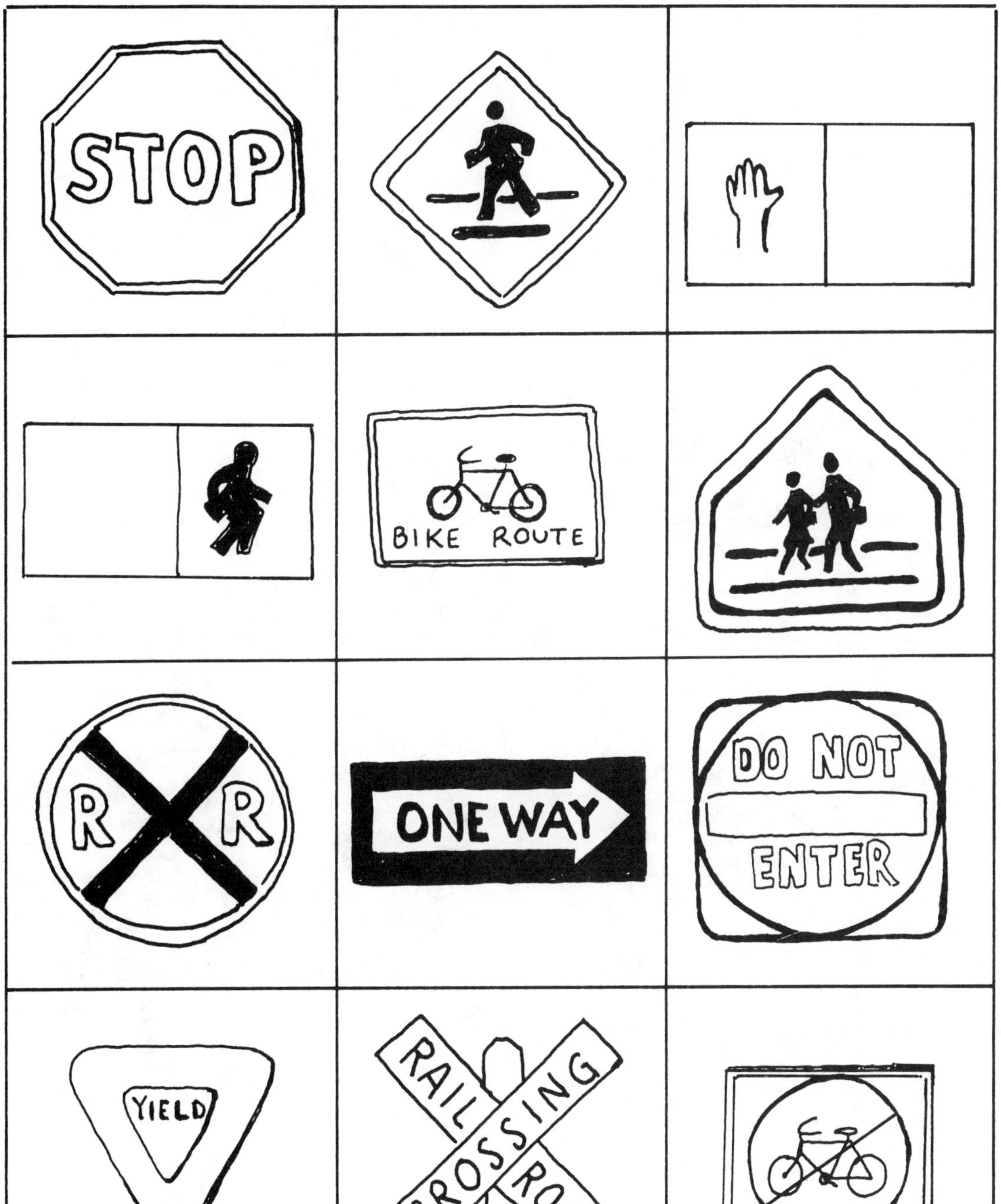

Name ______________________ Date ______________________

HIDDEN SIGNS

5–3A

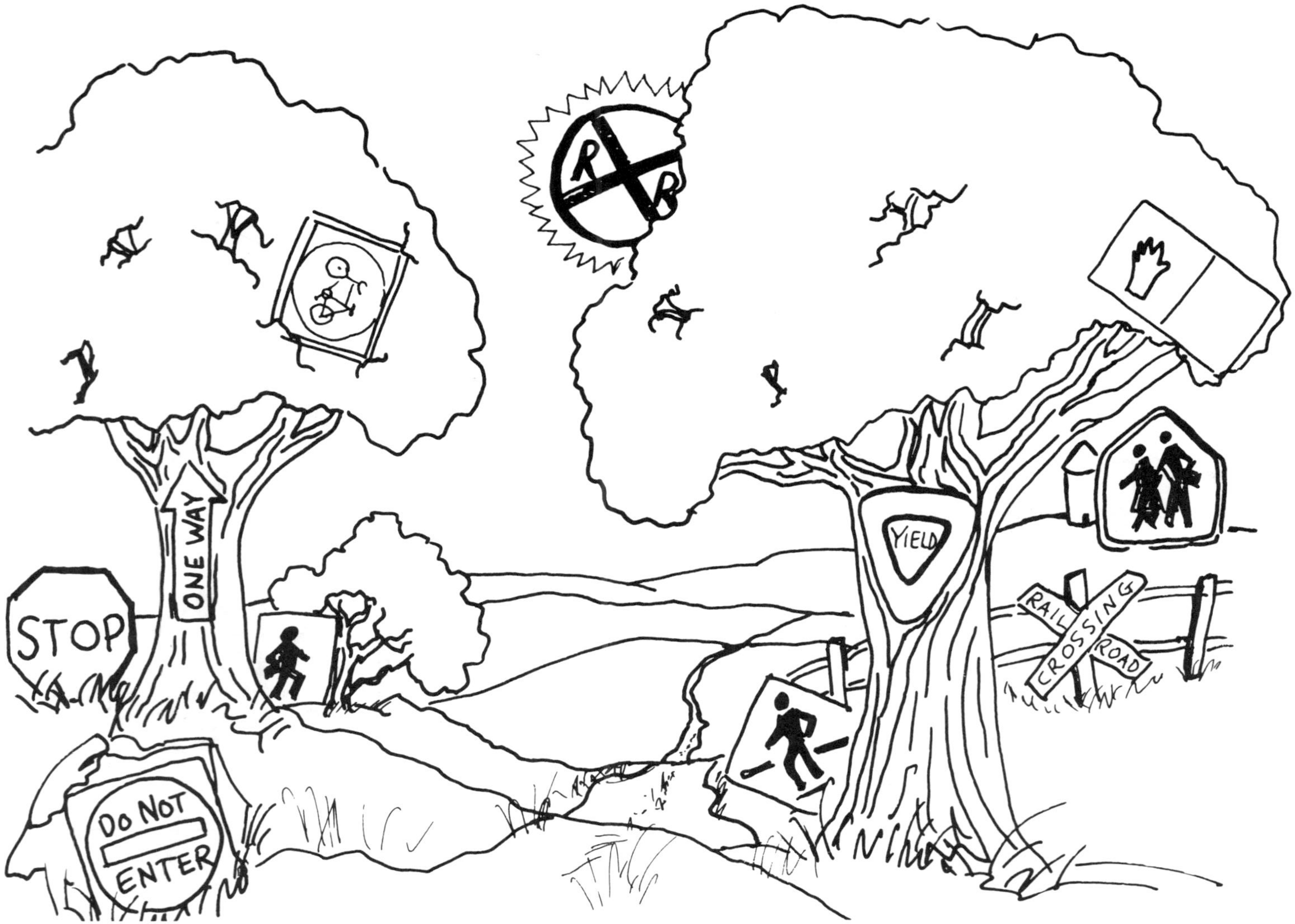

Name ______________________ Date ______________

SPIN-A-SIGN

5–4A

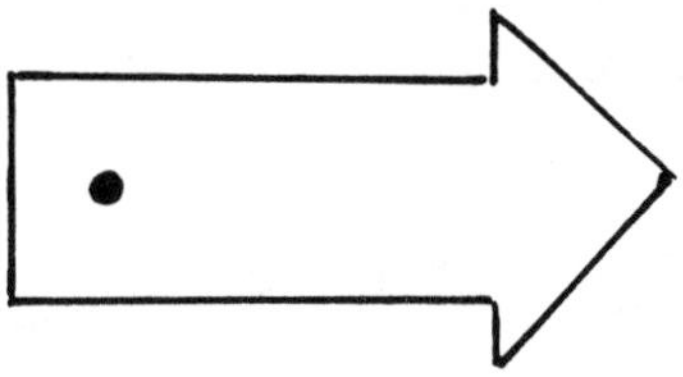

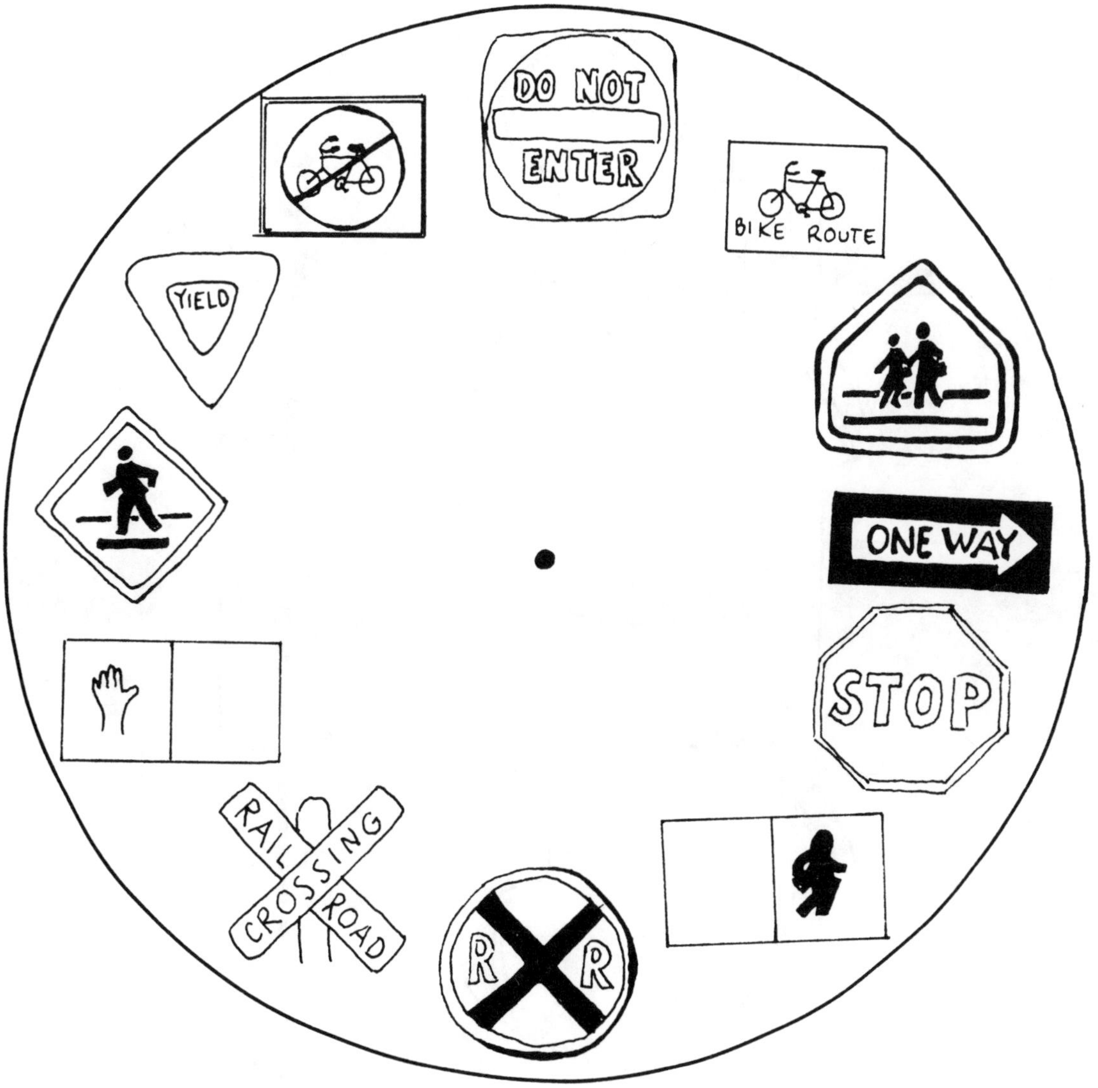

Name ____________________ Date ______________

TRAFFIC SIGNAL *5–5A*

Color the top light on the traffic signal red. Color the middle light yellow. Color the bottom light green. Explain to a friend what each light means.

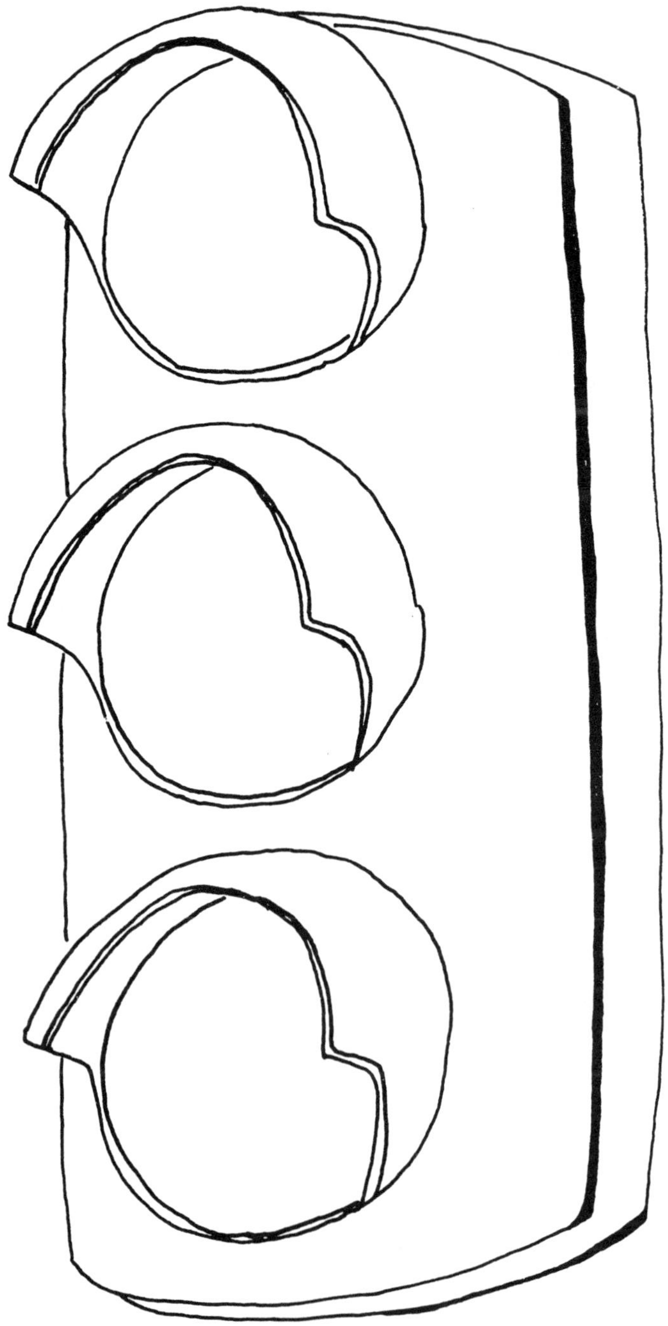

Name ______________________ Date ______________

EXIT SIGN *5–6A*

Always look for this sign when you go into a building. It tells you where the doors are. Look for the **EXIT** sign if you need to leave the building quickly.

Tear red paper into small pieces. Glue the pieces of paper to the letters.

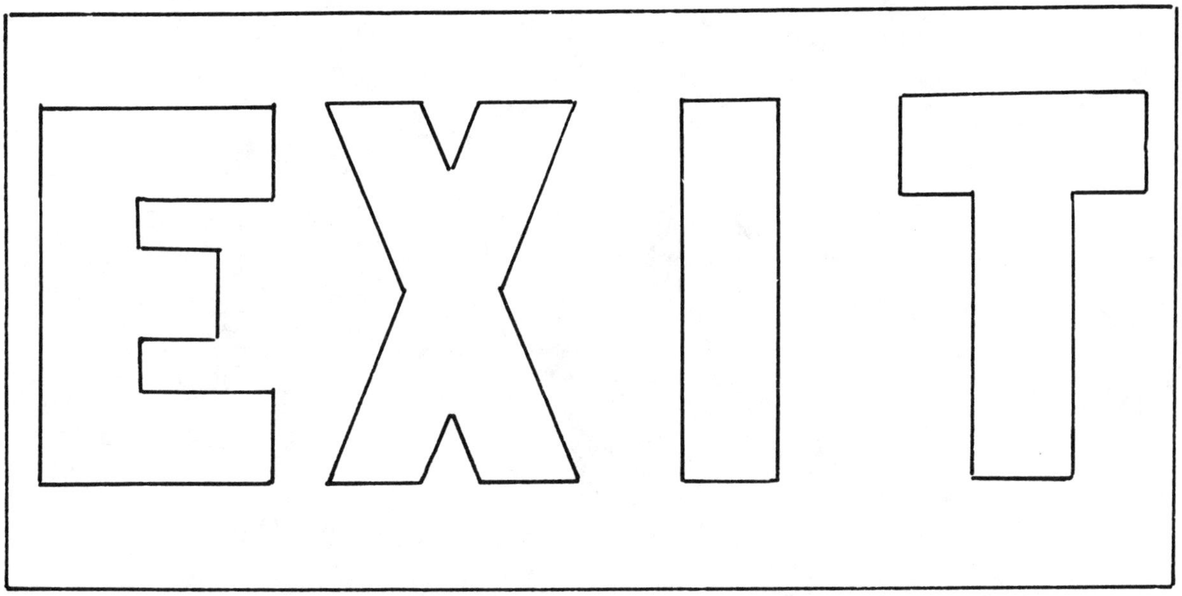

POISON PUZZLE

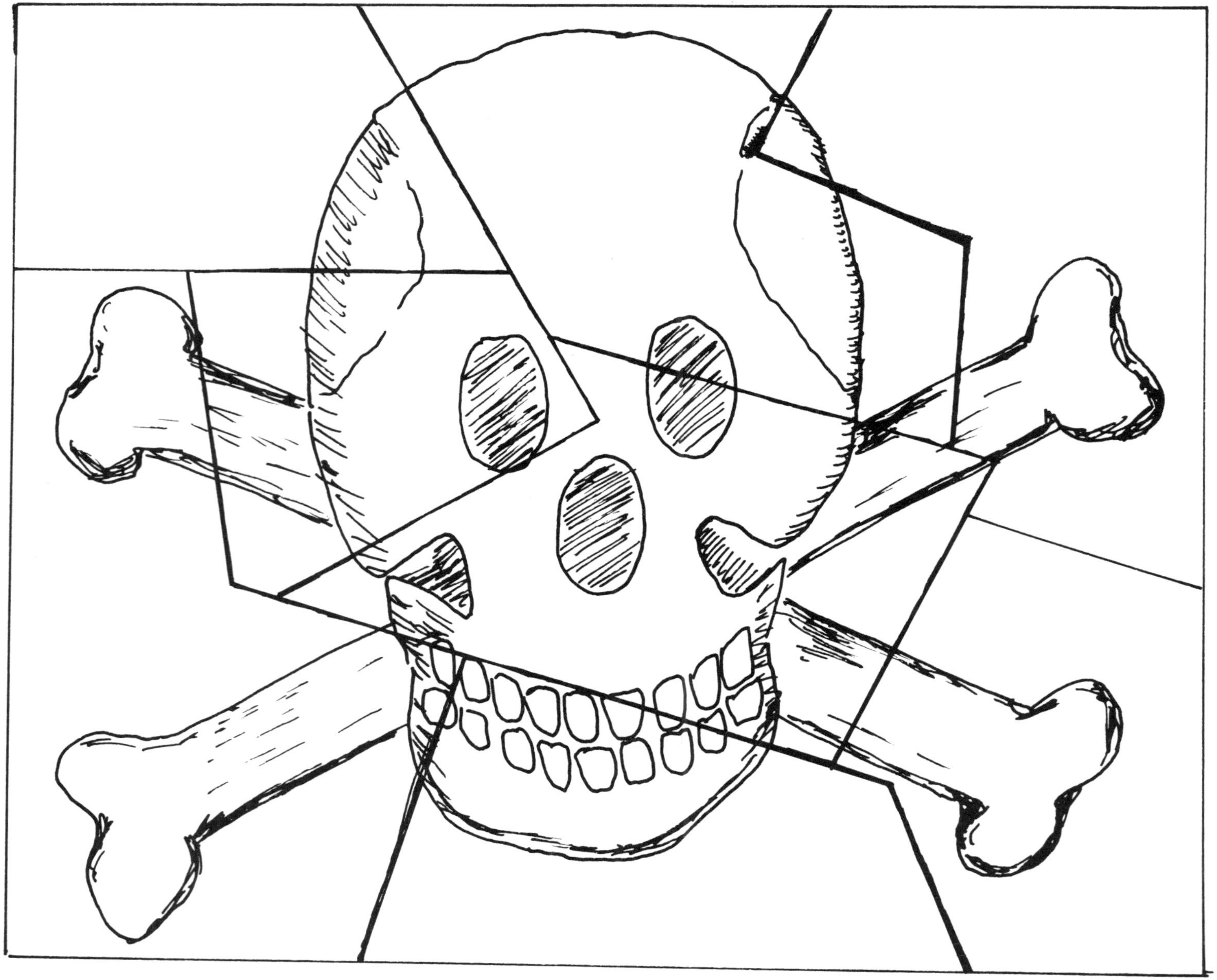

Name ______________________ Date ______________

SAFETY STORY 1

5–8A

 stayed at home while

Sean

his  went to the

mother

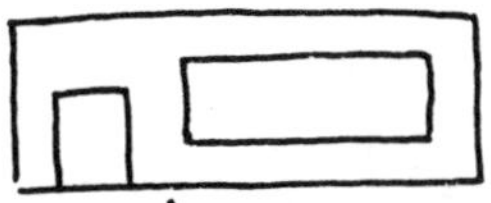 The 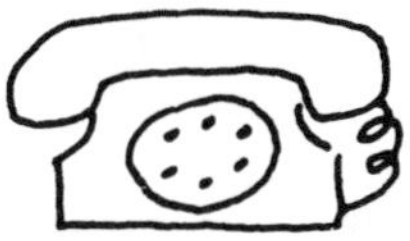 rang. When

store. phone

 answered, the caller

Sean

asked for Sean's 

mother.

What should Sean say?

____

____

____

____

Name ______________________ Date ______________

SAFETY STORY 2 ***5–8B***

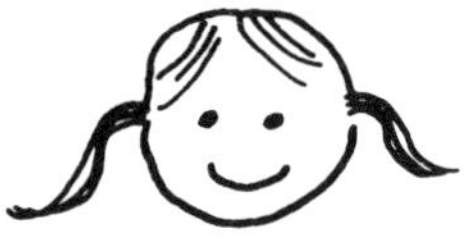 was home alone.
Emily

She heard a knock at the

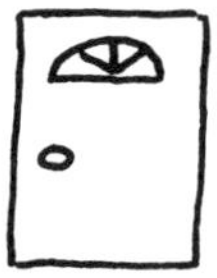  asked, "Who is
door. Emily

it?" The person at the 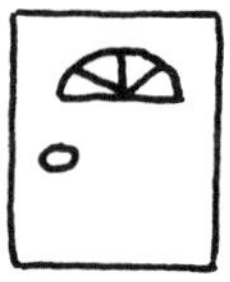
door

said, "I have a package for you."

What should Emily do?

____

____

____

____

Name ______________________ Date ______________

SAFETY STORY 3

5–8C

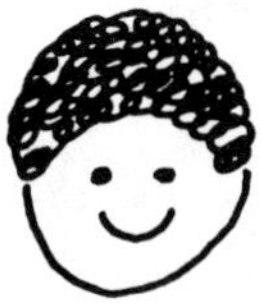 and 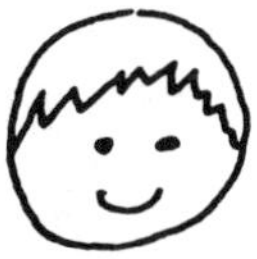 were
Megan Jacob

walking home from

School. A 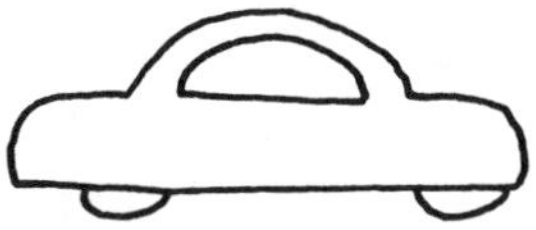 stopped.
car

The driver offered

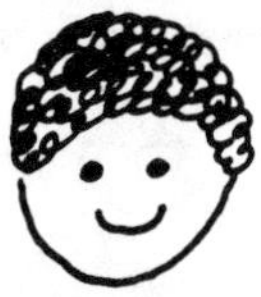 and 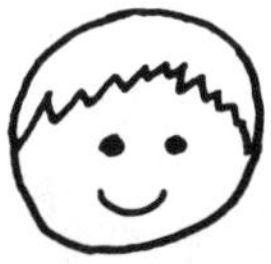 a ride.
Megan Jacob

What should they do?

____

____

____

____

Name ______________________ Date ______________

SAFETY STORY 4

5–8D

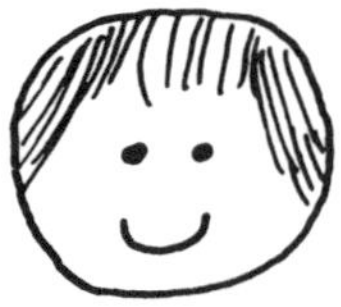
Jessica was playing with

her friends at the 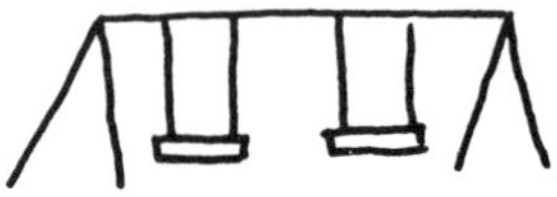
park.

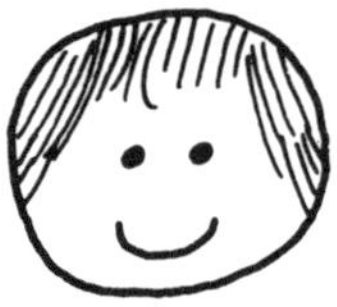
Jessica wanted to go home

but her friends wanted

to stay at the 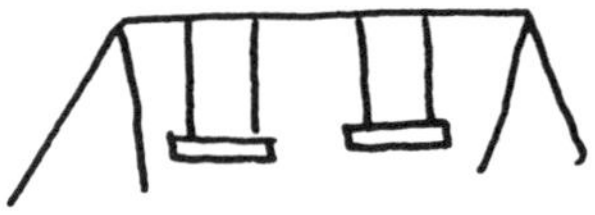
park.

What should Jessica do?

____

____

____

____

Name ______________________ Date ______________

BICYCLE SAFETY *5–9A*

Help Andrew get ready for a bike ride. Draw circles around things that will protect him as he rides. Put an X on each thing that is not safe to wear for bicycle riding.

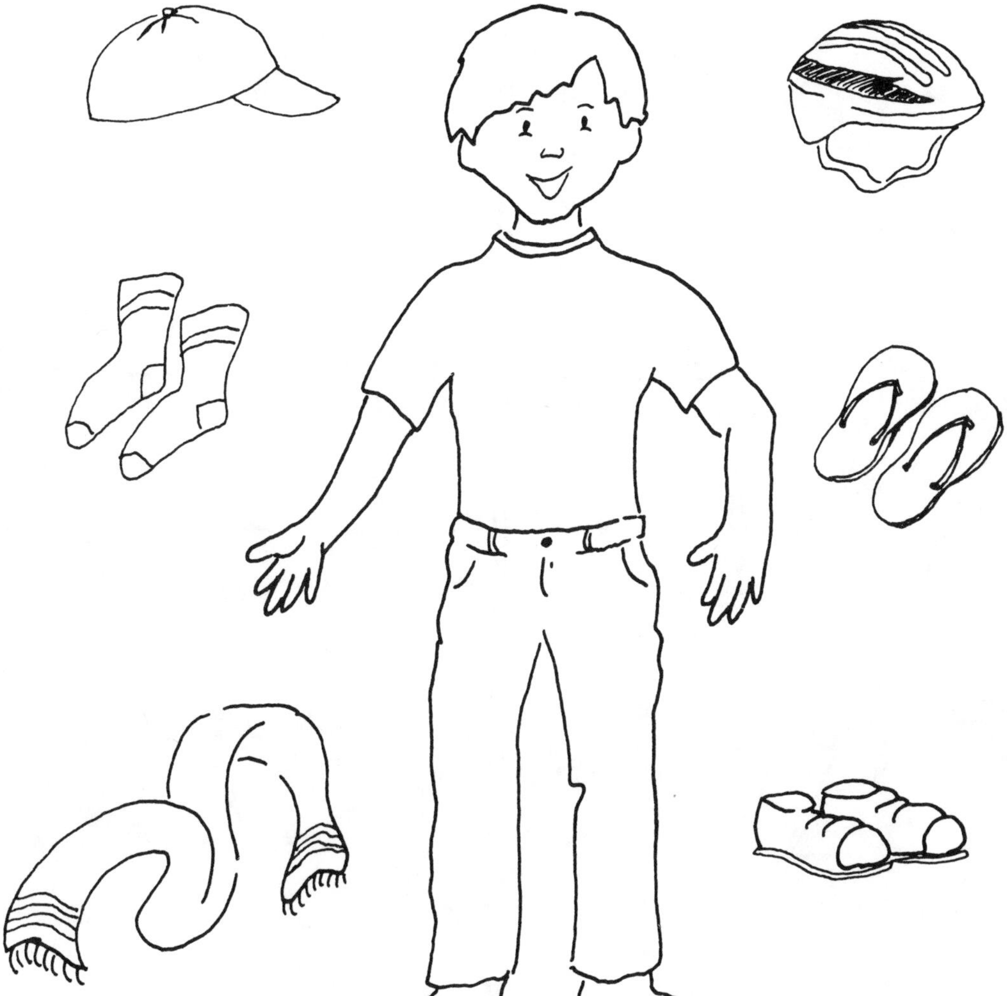

Name ______________________________ **Date** ____________________

KITE PATTERN *5–10A*

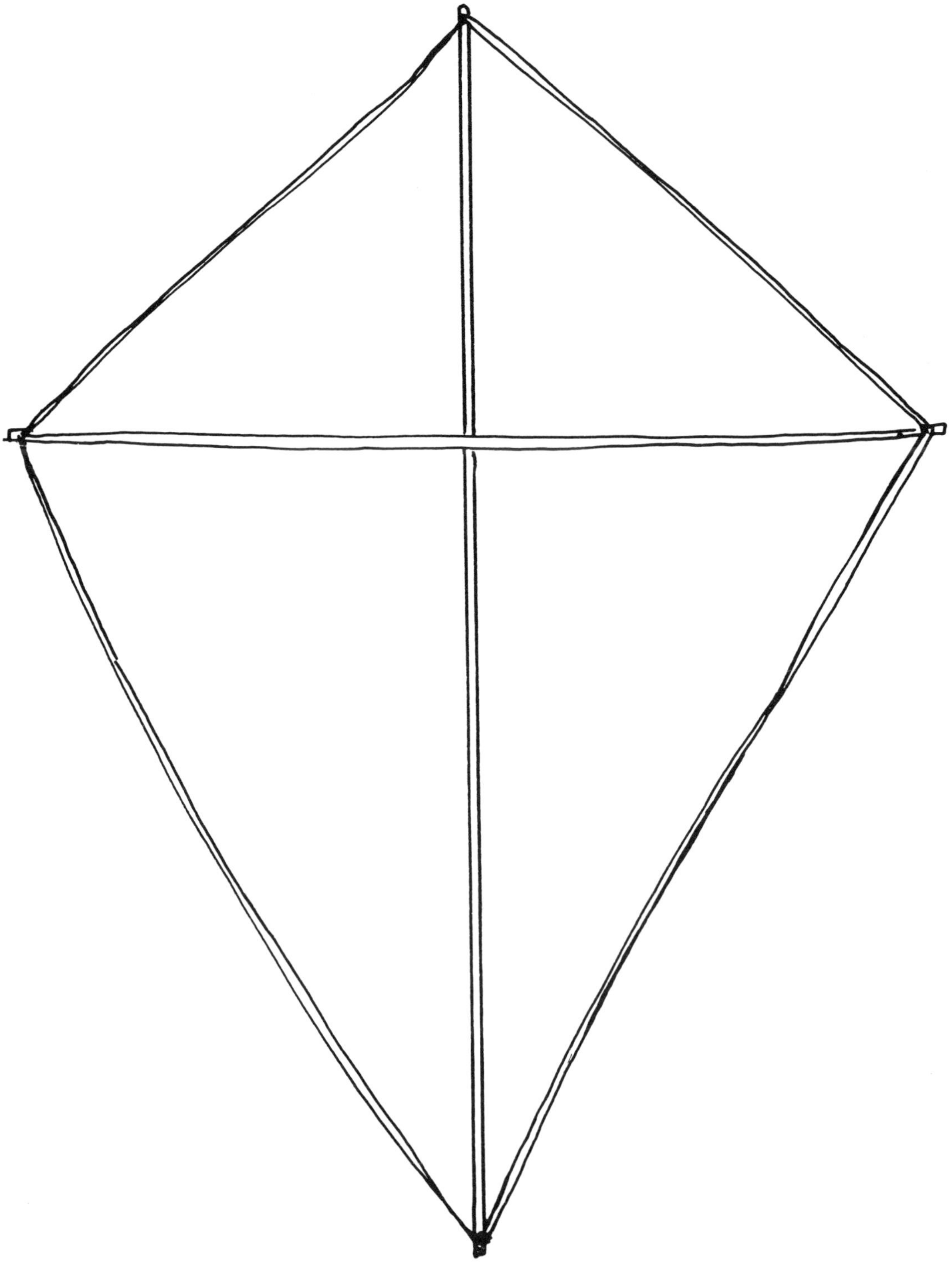

Name ______________________________ Date ______________

DO NOT TOUCH/HANDLE WITH CARE *5–11A*

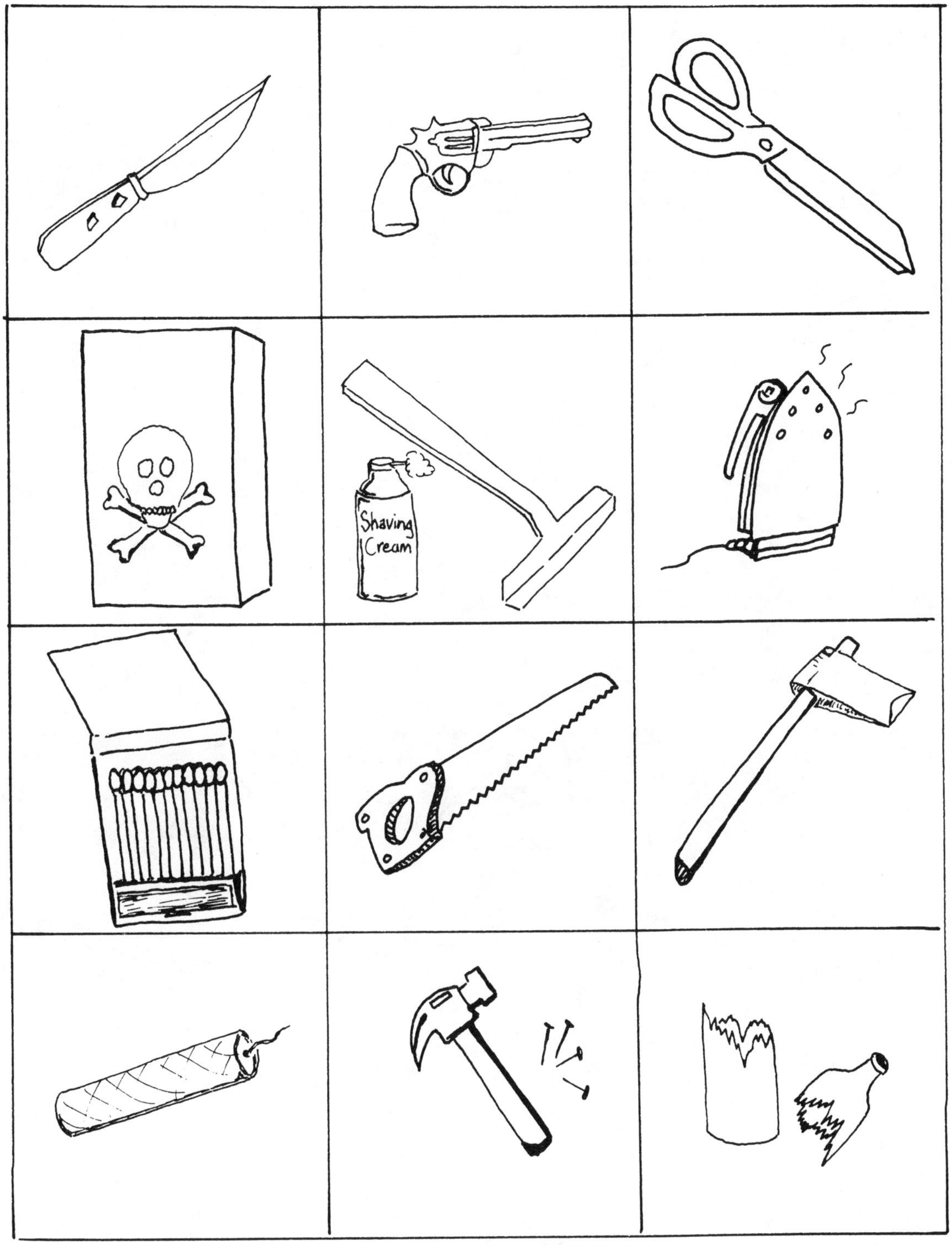

Name ______________________ Date ______________

INDOOR FIRE SAFETY *5–14A*

Start at the arrow and draw a line along the path. When you come to a place where a fire might start, put an X on it.

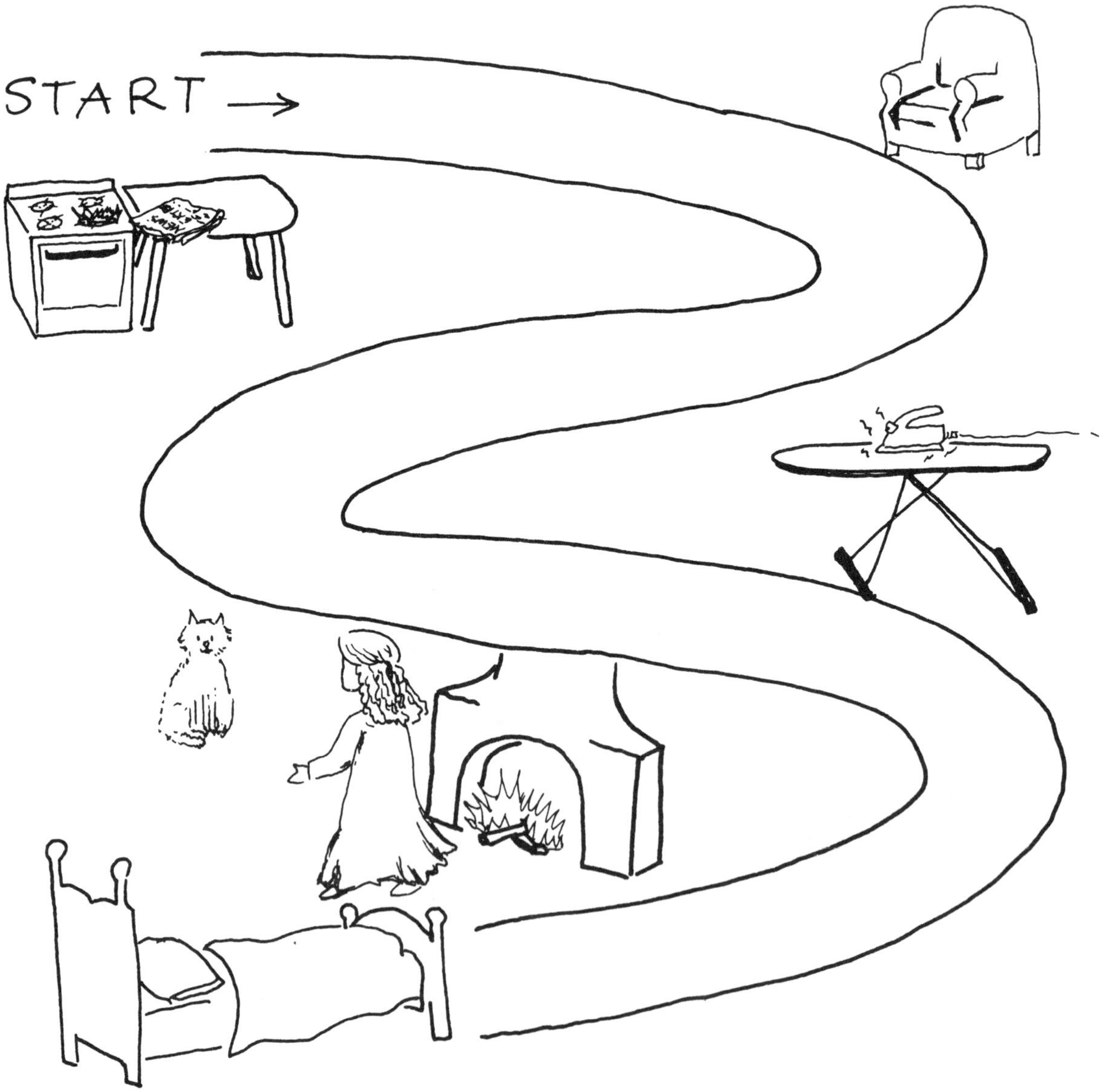

Name ______________________ Date ____________

OUTDOOR FIRE SAFETY *5–14B*

Start at the arrow and draw a line along the path. When you come to a place where a fire might start, put an X on it.

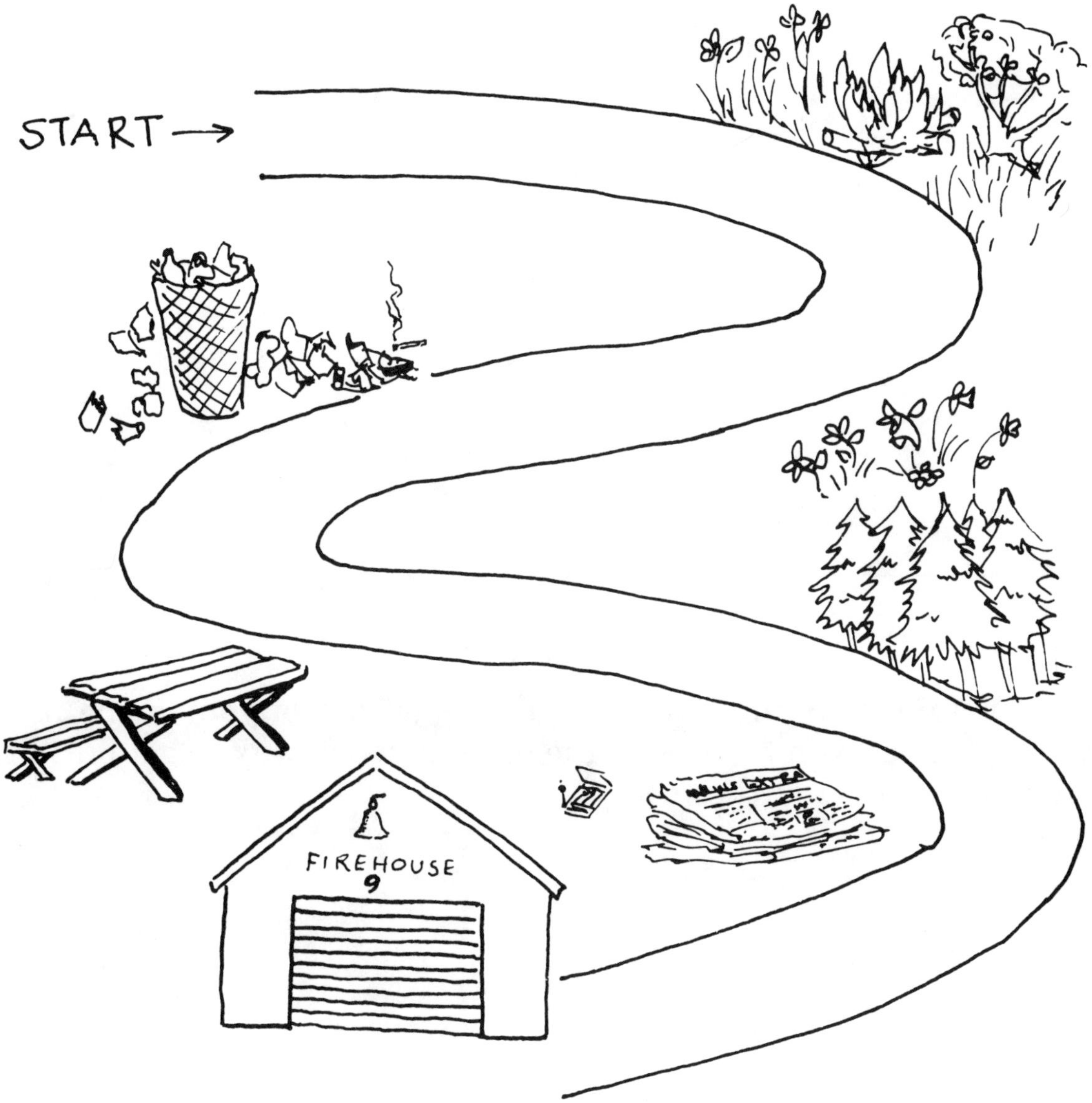

Name ______________________________ Date ________________

ESCAPE ROUTE *5–14C*

Pretend you are looking down through the roof of your home. Ask your family to help you draw a floor plan that shows where the rooms, the stairways, the windows, and the doors are.

Floor plan of my home

With your family, figure out two ways to get out of your home in case of fire. Use a red crayon to draw a line showing each way to get out. Practice leaving your home by those ways.

Fire safety questions:

Do you have smoke detectors at home? ☐ Yes ☐ No

Do your smoke detectors work? ☐ Yes ☐ No

Name ______________________________ Date ________________

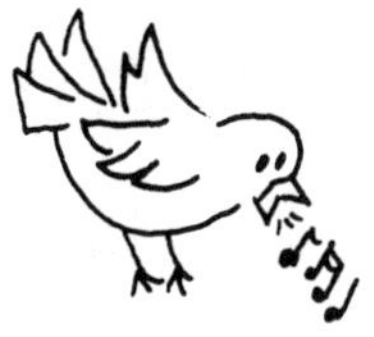

EMERGENCY NUMBER

5–15A

Write the numbers to push or dial when you need help in an emergency.

____

Color those buttons red on the telephone.

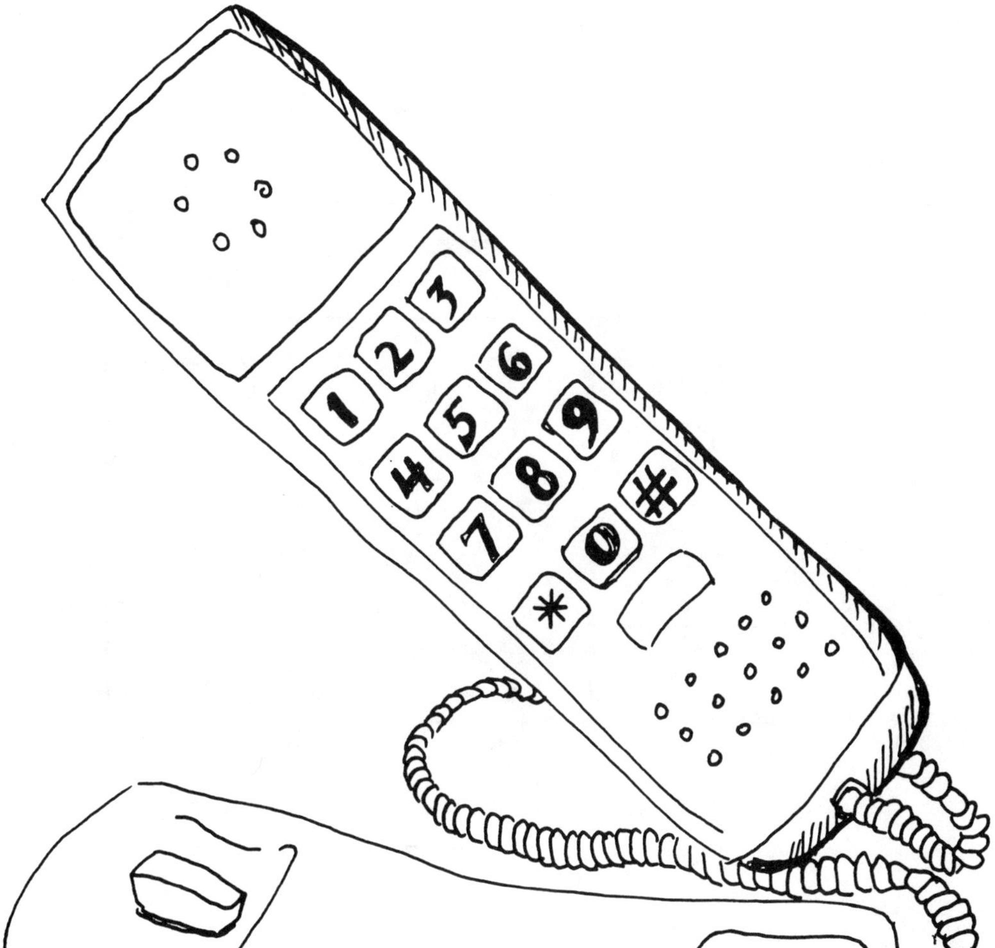

Name ______________________ Date ______________

SAFETY CODE *5–17A*

Look at the code at the top and write the letters in the same shapes below. Read the words to find out what to do if your clothes catch on fire.

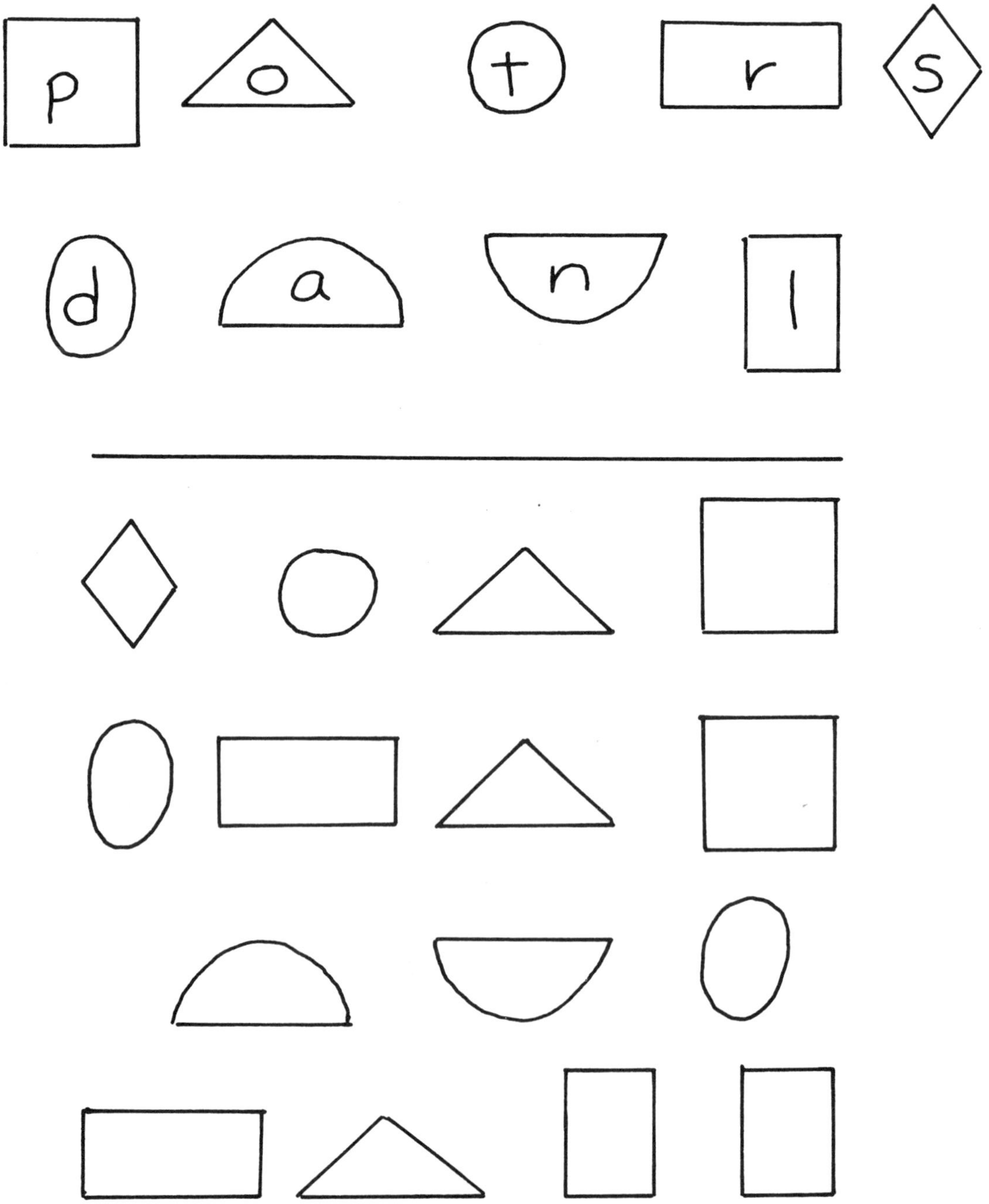

Name ________________________________ Date ________________

DRAW-A-SIGN *5–17B*

Draw the sign that warns you to watch out for trains.

Draw the sign that tells you to stop.

Draw the symbol that warns you about something that could make you very sick.

Draw the sign that shows you a safe place to ride your bike.

Draw the symbol that tells you not to cross the street.

Name ______________________________ Date ____________________

SAFETY PUZZLE *5–17C*

Cross out the first letter and then every other letter. Write the letters that are left in the blanks. Explain to a friend what each word means.

1. J E P X A I B T

_ _ _ _

2. X P Q O H I B S C O S N

_ _ _ _ _ _

3. D S K T Z R A A W N U G M E E R

_ _ _ _ _ _ _ _

4. B S O T A O X P

_ _ _ _

5. P E T M A E N R D G I E X N D C O Y

_ _ _ _ _ _ _ _ _

6. O S R A W F G E P T H Y

_ _ _ _ _ _

6 — EXERCISE

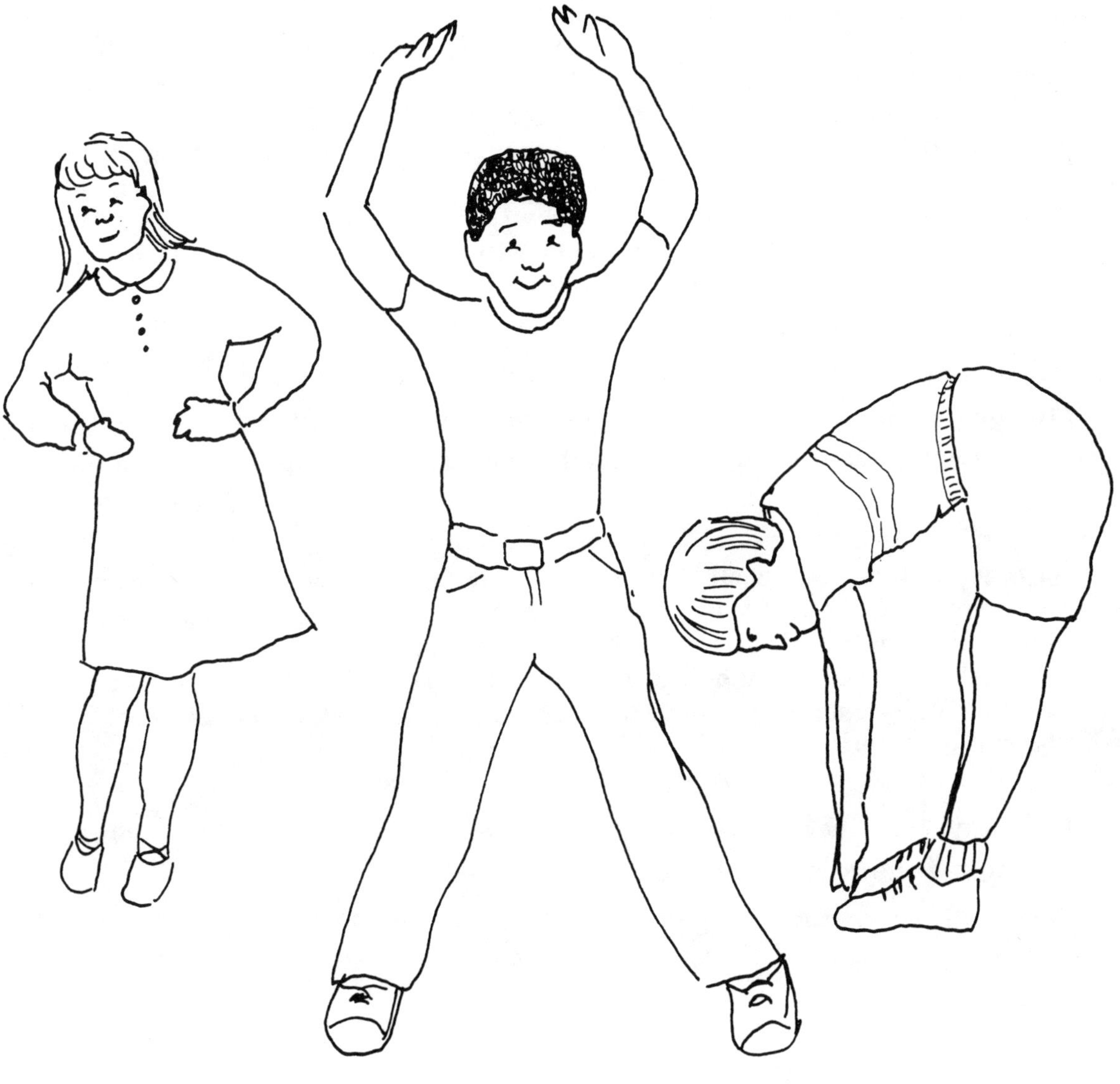

Exercising and being physically active are important for good health. By encouraging your students to actively participate in physical fitness activities, you can influence their health now and in the future. Exercise helps children feel and look better. According to the American Heart Association, exercise can also reduce stress, help build physical strength and stamina, improve circulation, and enable the heart and lungs to function more efficiently. Physical fitness and academic achievement often go hand in hand.

Studies show that the level of physical fitness is declining among today's children. In general, according to pediatricians and fitness experts, children today are more sedentary and obese than previous generations. Large numbers of children are not able to meet fitness standards in tests designed to measure lower back flexibility, abdominal muscle tone, upper body strength, and cardiovascular fitness.

The exercises in this section are designed to increase children's physical fitness while they engage in interesting, enjoyable activities. In order to be effective, children and adults must exercise on a regular basis. For this reason, try to schedule physical fitness activities every day.

It is important to begin each exercise session with a five-minute warm-up period. See Warm Up, Cool Down (activity 6–1) for warm-up suggestions, or demonstrate the following movements and have students repeat them five times:

- stand and swing both arms slowly forward, and then backward;
- stand and pull each knee toward the chest;
- stand on your toes and then drop slowly back to your heels;
- stand and grasp hands above your head. Bend slowly first to the right and then to the left.

After each exercise session, have students walk around and cool down for about five minutes.

In order to avoid injury, have children stretch and bend slowly and easily. Show them how to bend their knees when doing toe touches, situps, or leg lifts. Avoid any exercises that involve heavy lifting or pulling and those that might pull or strain muscles.

Several review sheets are included at the end of the Exercise section. These sheets reinforce the message that daily exercise is important; they may be used as independent activities or placed in learning centers.

The activities in the Exercise section will help students:

- understand that exercise and physical fitness are important parts of being healthy;
- begin to make exercise part of their daily routines;
- improve physical fitness, reduce stress, and increase physical strength and stamina;
- participate in a variety of enjoyable physical fitness activities.

6–1 WARM UP, COOL DOWN

Stretching and warming up before exercising help prevent body injuries.

This easy warm-up activity will help students get ready for other exercises. Read the poem aloud and have the students do the motions:

Shake fingers and toesies
Then tickle your knees.
Take a deep breath
And sway with the breeze.
Shake elbows and shoulders.
Stretch out, everyone.
Stretch your whole body
And reach for the sun.
Shake elbows and shoulders
And wiggle your feet
Then shake your whole body
And strut down the street.

Stretching and cooling down after exercising help muscles stay healthy. Read the poem aloud and have the students do the motions:

Take a deep breath now
And stretch out in space.
Then stretch your whole body.
Sit down in your place.

6–2 GET UP AND GO!

Exercising every day is essential for promoting good physical and mental health. The four activities in this exercise course will encourage sedentary children to do more physical movement.

Materials:

masking tape

scissors

copies of Fitness Signs pages 6–2A and 6–2B

Directions:

Cut each Fitness Sign page apart to make four Fitness Signs. Show the Fitness Signs one at a time. Read the directions for each exercise aloud. Show how to do each exercise and have students do it with you.

BREATHE DEEPLY

Stand tall. Take a deep breath as you rise on your toes and slowly move your arms in a circle inward and upward. Hold your arms overhead to a count of five, then slowly circle them to the side and down as you lower your heels and let out your breath. Slowly count to five each time you do the breathing exercise.

RUN IN PLACE

Stand tall. Pump your arms, raise your knees as high as you can, and run without moving forward. Count each time your left foot touches the floor. See if you can run for 30 counts. Stop and rest if you are tired.

LEFT HAND/RIGHT HAND TOE TOUCH

Stand tall with your knees slightly bent and legs spread widely apart. Bend at the waist, keep your arms straight and touch your right hand to your left toes. Come back to your starting position. Bend your waist, keep your arms straight and touch your left hand to your right toes. Come back to your starting position.

JUMPING JACKS

Stand tall with your arms at your sides and your feet together. Raise your arms overhead and touch your hands together as you jump and spread your feet apart sideways. Bring your hands back to your sides as you jump and bring your feet together again. Do ten jumping jacks.

After demonstrating the exercises, tape the signs in various places around the room. Have the students line up single file and walk from sign to sign. Tell them to do the exercise shown on each sign. Leave the signs in place and have students use the exercise course every day.

Give each of the students a set of Fitness Stations signs. Encourage them to make an exercise course at home and ask family members to exercise with them each day.

6–3 EXERCISE EVERY DAY

Encourage students to get into the habit of exercising every day.

Materials:

copies of Exercise Wheel 6–3A
copies of Exercise Chart 6–3B
scissors
9″ paper plates
glue
pencils
paper fasteners

Preparation:

1. Cut out the circle and arrow from one Exercise Wheel page.
2. Glue the Exercise Wheel to a paper plate.
3. Line up the black dots on the arrow and the Exercise Wheel. Push a pencil point through both dots to make an opening. Attach the arrow to the Exercise Wheel with a paper fastener.

Directions:

Distribute an Exercise Wheel page, a paper plate, and a paper fastener to each student. Help students assemble their Exercise Wheels, following the directions in "Preparation."

Afterwards, show your Exercise Wheel and move the arrow to point to each exercise, one by one. Have students move the arrows on their Exercise Wheels to point to the same exercise. Read the directions for each exercise aloud. Show how to do each one and have students do it with you.

JUMPING JACKS

Stand tall with your arms at your sides and your feet together. Raise your arms overhead and touch your hands together as you jump and spread your feet apart sideways. Bring your hands back to your sides as you jump and bring your feet together again. Do ten jumping jacks.

RUN IN PLACE

Stand tall. Pump your arms, raise your knees as high as you can, and run without moving forward. Count each time your left foot touches the floor. See if you can run for 30 counts. Stop and rest if you are tired.

TOUCH YOUR TOES

Stand tall with your knees bent and your feet slightly apart. Raise your arms above your head, and then slowly bend forward and reach toward your toes with your fingertips. Slowly straighten up and raise your arms overhead again. Repeat five times.

LEG LIFTS

Lie on your back on the floor. Bend your left leg at the knee. Slowly raise your right leg as high as you can. Hold it high while you count to five, and then slowly lower it again. Then bend your right leg at the knee and lift your left leg. Lift each leg five times.

Have students take their Exercise Wheels home, and encourage them to invite family members to exercise with them every day.

Display your Exercise Wheel in the classroom. Each day, let one student move the arrow to point to one of the four exercises shown, and then lead the rest of the class in doing the exercise he or she has chosen.

Give each of the students an Exercise Chart to add to their "Here's to My Health" booklet file folders. Tell them to color a space on the chart each time they exercise.

6–4 STRETCHERS

Using a plastic coil toy is a simple way to exercise hands and arms.

Materials:

plastic coil toy

Directions:

Let each student take a turn doing these arm-stretching movements. Give these instructions:

1. Hold one end of the toy in each hand and stretch your arms out to the side as far as you can.
2. Raise your arms overhead and stretch the toy as far to each side as you can.
3. Hold the toy behind your back and stretch it to the sides as far as you can.
4. Bend over forwards and stretch the toy to the sides as far as you can.
5. Hold one end of the toy on the floor with your left foot and pull the other end up as high as you can with your right hand.
6. Hold one end of the toy on the floor with your right foot and pull the other end up as high as you can with your left hand.

6–5 EXERCISING FUN, FUN, FUN

Exercise makes the body feel refreshed and lively.

Have the students remove their shoes and sit on the floor a space apart. Read the poem aloud and tell the students to act out the motions.

Do you suppose?
Do you suppose
Your left, left foot can touch your nose?
Now won't you try?
Now won't you try
Your right, right foot up by your eye?
Please let me see.
Please let me see.
Your left, left elbow touch your knee.
Oh, here you go.
Oh, here you go.
Your right, right elbow near a toe.
Then show me please.
Then show me please
If your head can touch your knees.
Touch hands and feet
And then you're done
With exercising fun, fun, fun.

6–6 ROLL-ALONG ROAD

This road-rolling exercise is good for developing coordination skills.

Materials:

skateboard
scooter

Preparation:

Chalk or tape a short winding roadway on the floor or playground. Put a starting line at one end and a finish line at the other.

Directions:

Ask the students to line up single file at the starting line. Have them take turns balancing face down on their stomachs on a skateboard. Tell them to push on the ground with their hands and slowly move the skateboard forward. Have them see if they can roll to the finish line without going off the road.

When everyone has had a turn have them repeat the exercise using a scooter.

Have the students use the Roll-Along Road each week. Ask the students to see if they can go a longer distance each time they use the Roll-Along Road. Ask if they can think of something else they could use on the road.

Encourage students to make a Roll-Along Road at home or in the park. Tell them to practice using it everyday with a skateboard or scooter.

6–7 SQUEEZE A BALL

Hands need to be exercised to strengthen muscles.

Materials:

small rubber ball

Directions:

Have the students sit in a circle on the floor. Pass a small rubber ball around the circle to the right. Ask each student to squeeze the ball hard with the right hand then pass it to the person on their right. When the ball is back where it started have the student squeeze the ball hard with the left hand and pass it to the person on their left.

Ask the students to describe how their hands felt when they squeezed the ball. Ask: "Did you feel your muscles working when you squeezed the ball?"

6–8 TENSION TAKERS

Help chase tensions away with these slow exercises.

Directions:

Show the students how to inhale and exhale properly by lying on their backs and closing their mouths. Tell them to take a deep breath through the nostrils then open their mouths and slowly blow out the air with a hissing sound. Tell them to breathe this way while doing the exercises. Ask the students to take a short rest between each exercise if they feel any pain.

1. Tell the students to lie flat on the floor on their backs with their arms at their sides and toes pointed up. Ask them to inhale and stretch their arms up over their heads. Have them continue stretching as they inhale, and then slowly put their arms down and relax for a short time. Repeat three times.
2. Ask the students to sit comfortably on the floor and relax their shoulders. Have them roll their shoulders slowly to the front three times and then to the back three times.
3. Have the students sit up straight on the floor. Tell them to take a deep breath and blow it out, then slowly move their head towards their right shoulder as you count to ten. Have them repeat the exercise, moving their head towards the left shoulder.
4. Ask the students to sit straight and move both shoulders up towards their ears as you count to five. Have them lower their shoulders as far as they can as you count to five. Ask them to roll their shoulders forward without hunching their backs as you count to five. Then have them push their shoulders back and squeeze their shoulder blades together as you count to five.

6–9 JACK-IN-THE-BOX

Read the poem aloud, emphasizing the underlined words. Tell the students to listen to the poem and do the motions:

Jack-in-the-Box
When you hear <u>one</u>
Curl up for
Some special fun.
Jack-in-the-Box,
When you hear <u>two</u>
Close your eyes
And touch your shoe.
Jack-in-the-Box,
When you hear <u>three</u>
Put a hand
On each knee.
Jack-in-the-Box,
When you hear <u>four</u>
Stretch your arms.
Touch the floor.
Jack-in-the-Box,
When you hear <u>five</u>
Pop up high
And come alive!!

6–10 MOVE FOR A MINUTE

Many movements can be done in a minute.

Materials:

stopwatch or watch with a second hand

Directions:

Read the poem aloud and tell the students to move for a minute. Time the activity with a stopwatch.

Move for a minute.
Ready, set, go.
Wiggle your body.
Let yourself flow.

Move for a minute.
Sway in the sun.
Kick up your heels.
Smile and have fun.

Move for a minute.
Bend in the breeze.
Jump in a circle.
Tickle your knees.

Move for a minute.
Shake and shout.
Jiggle your elbows.
Twist about.

Move for a minute.
Stretch out far
Try to catch
A shooting star.

Move for a minute.
Spin around.
March and make
An oompah sound.

Move for a minute.
Run in place.
Dance your fingers
Out in space.

Move for a minute
How you like best.
Then stop and take
A one-minute rest.

6–11 SHAKE THE SHEET

Everybody will have fun as they exercise their arms in this group activity.

Materials:

an old sheet
two or three beach balls

Directions:

Spread the sheet on the floor. Group the students around the sheet. Have them pick up the sheet and hold it tightly at waist level with both hands. Put the beach balls on the sheet and have the students shake the sheet trying not to let the balls roll off it.

6–12 FOOT WORK

Feet need to be exercised every day to stay healthy.

Materials:

marbles
pencil
small ball
chair

Directions:

Have the students take off their shoes and lie on their backs with their legs straight out in front of them. Have them shake their feet a little, then point their toes toward their heads, heels pointing out. Tell them to slowly stretch their toes forward. Have them do the exercise three times and then shake their feet.

Ask the students to lie on their backs facing a partner. Tell them to put their feet against their partner's feet and slowly push back and forth. Have them raise their feet higher and move them faster.

Have the students take off their socks. Put several marbles on the floor in front of a chair. Have the students sit down and take turns trying to pick up a marble between their toes.

Tell them to gently roll the marbles under their feet. Then ask them how it feels.

Put a pencil and a small ball on the floor and have the students roll them with their feet. Ask how it feels to roll the pencil and ball.

6–13 EVERYBODY JOIN THE GYM

It's fun to sing and get in shape at the same time.

Ask the students to form a large circle and stand a few feet apart. Have them slowly sing this song to the tune of "Old MacDonald Had a Farm," and do the exercises mentioned:

Everybody join the gym.
Ei-igh-ee-igh-oh.
And in that gym we'll exercise.
Ei-igh-ee-igh-oh.
With a shake, shake here
And a shake, shake there.
Here a shake,
There a shake,
Everywhere a shake, shake.
Everybody join the gym.
Ei-igh-ee-igh-ohhhhh.

Use the words shake, stretch, hop, skip, jump, kick, bend, tiptoe and shake again.

6–14 FLAP YOUR WINGS, BIRDIES

This exercise will help improve posture and strengthen shoulder and arm muscles.

Ask the students to stand straight with their feet a few feet apart. Have them raise their elbows in front even with their shoulders. Tell them to push their arms to their sides.

Read the poem aloud and have the students continue chanting it as they flap their arms like wings and fly around.

Flap your wings, birdies,
And fly away.
Fly around on
This beautiful day.

After awhile say:

Fly away, birdies,
Home to your nests.
Fold your wings, birdies,
And take a rest.

Have the students fly home to where they started and rest on the floor.

6–15 MENU MOVEMENT

Favorite foods and movement combine to make a fun activity. Read the poem aloud and have the students do the actions:

If you like apples
Run in your own place.
If you like baked potatoes
Walk in outer space.
If you like cantaloupe
Do a dance that's slow.
If you like green beans
Kick up your left toe.
If you like pasta
Fly away to Mars.
If you like chicken
Reach for shooting stars.
If you like bananas
Climb a shady tree.
If you like carrots
Jiggle your right knee.
If you like yogurt
Wiggle all your clothes.
If you like tortillas
Tickle all your toes.
If you like corn on the cob
Count by two's to ten.
Two, four, six, eight, ten.
Do the poem again.

6–16 SKY DANCING

Fingers and toes need exercise as much as the rest of the body.

Materials:

record player or cassette player
records or cassettes

Directions:

Ask the students to take off their shoes and lie down a space apart. Play some dancing music for the students. Read the poem aloud and have the students act out the sky dancing motions:

Fingers out. Fingers out
Far as they can go.
Fingers up. Fingers up
Standing in a row.
Fingers close. Fingers close
Waiting for the chance
To open up, open up
In a graceful dance.
Toes go up. Toes go up
Far as they can go.
Toes point up. Toes point up
Standing in a row.
Make them swirl. Make them sway
Up, up, up so high
Toes and fingers dancing now,
Dancing in the sky.

6–17 HAND DANCING

Hands moving to music is an enjoyable way to exercise.

Materials:

record player or cassette player
records or cassettes

Directions:

Have each student sit on the floor facing a partner. Tell them to spread their fingers wide and press them against their partner's fingers. Put on some music and ask the students to do "hand dancing" in the air. Have them try one-handed dancing with a partner. Ask them to shake their hands in the air and then do their hand dancing alone.

6–18 HANDS AND FINGERS

Exercising hands and fingers keeps them flexible.

Have the students sit on the floor in a circle. Read the poem aloud and have them do the motions:

Shake your fingers.
Hang them loose.
Wiggle them around.
Shake your fingers
Side to side then
Rest them on the ground.

Chalk a small circle, square, triangle and rectangle in front of each student. Ask them to take a "finger walk" along the lines.

Ask the students to spread their fingers wide. Have them press one hand against the other hand with palms out. Ask them to repeat the exercise a few times, then shake their fingers.

Tell the students to open and close their hands as many times as they can. Ask how their hands felt while they were opening and closing them. Tell them to try doing the exercise fast and slow. Have them shake their hands in the air and then fold and rest them on their laps.

6–19 SPIN AROUND

Have the students sit on the floor several feet away from their neighbor. Read the poem aloud and ask the students to follow the directions.

Sit on the floor.
Bend your legs.
Knees up to your chin.
Hold your arms
Around your legs.
Ready now . . . begin.
Spin around.
Spin around.
Spin around some more
Then arms out wide,
Legs out wide.
Spread out on the floor.

6–20 PEDAL PUSHING

Riding an imaginary bicycle in the air helps strengthen hip, lower back and leg muscles.

Have the students lie down on their backs several feet away from their neighbors. Read the poem aloud and have the students do the motions:

Feet high in the air.
Climb on your bike.
Go pedal pushing
Wherever you like.
Ride on the bike path
With some of your friends.
Riding along to
Where the path ends.
Stop for a rest now
Then finish your play
Riding your bicycle
Off and away!

6–21 TAKE A WALK

Walking is a wonderful way to exercise the whole body and get fresh air.

Read the poem aloud. Ask the students to do the motions:

Take a walk in the city
Down the busy streets.
Head up high. Swing your arms.
Move those busy feet.

Climb the stairs in a building
To the second floor.
Turn around. Step back down.
Hurry out the door.

Take a walk through the park.
See the sights and then
Move those feet. Cross the street.
Come back home again.

6–22 CATERPILLAR CRAWL-ALONG

Caterpillar crawl-along exercises the whole body.

Have the students take off their shoes and lie on their stomachs with arms and legs stretched out straight.

Read the poem aloud and ask the students to crawl across the room like caterpillars.

Do the caterpillar crawl
And pull yourselves about.
Put your backs up in the air
Then spread yourselves way out.

Do the caterpillar crawl.
Make your bodies bend.
Fast or slow, away you go
With caterpillar friends.

6–23 WORD WALK

Chalk the word EXERCISE in large letters about 12 inches apart on the floor. Put an arrow at the bottom of the first E and a finish line a few inches from the bottom of the last E.

Spell out and say the word to the students. Ask them to line up single file a few feet away from the word. Tell them they are going to each take a turn walking around the word. When the first student in line finishes walking the first letter have him or her jump to the X. Have the next student start walking. Have the students return to the starting place. Repeat the exercise with everyone carefully walking the word backwards.

When the students have finished walking the word backwards, ask them to spell the word and say it aloud.

6–24 LEAP THE LAKE

Legs and feet will be exercised in this jumping activity.

Materials:

string or yarn

Directions:

Place two pieces of string or yarn on the floor or playground parallel to each other and about 12 inches apart. Have the students line up along the side of one string. Tell them to jump across the "lake." When everyone has leaped across the lake, move one string 3 inches farther away and have the students jump again. Continue widening the lake 3 inches each time until it is too wide to jump across.

6–25 ALLIGATOR IN THE LAKE

Use this running and leaping activity to exercise legs and feet.

Materials:

large brown paper grocery bag
beanbag

Directions:

Chalk a line on the floor or playground. Put the beanbag in the paper bag and place it about 15 feet away from the line. Tell the students it is a sleeping alligator who might wake up at any time. Have the students line up single file behind the line. Read the poem aloud and have the students chant it as they run one at a time and leap over the bag.

Alligator, alligator,
Please stay asleep.
Don't wake up
When I run and leap.

Tell the students to line up again when everyone has had a turn. See if they can leap higher on their second leap.

6–26 SOMERSAULTS

Ask the students to sit on the floor or playground and take off their shoes.

Have a few students at a time spread out a space apart and do some somersaults on a soft surface.

Read the poem aloud:

Somersaults, somersaults,
How many can you do?
Each time you roll over
Count one somersault for you.

6–27 BALANCE YOUR BODY

A slow motion exercise to help develop balancing skills.

Materials:

masking tape
shoe box lid
beanbag
feather
4 yardsticks

Directions:

Cut strips of masking tape to form a large square, circle, rectangle and triangle on the floor. Have the students take off their shoes and form a single line. Place the yardsticks on the floor end to end. Give these instructions:

1. When it is your turn, walk slowly around each shape and then return to the row.
2. When your turn comes again, place a shoe box lid on the palm of your hand and repeat the exercise.
3. Repeat the exercise with a beanbag.
4. Repeat the exercise with a feather.
5. Hold your arms out to the side and walk carefully along the yardsticks trying not to fall off.

6–28 FITNESS FUN

Daily exercise is necessary to help the body stay healthy. These hoop exercises are fun and will help students keep fit.

Materials:

several large plastic hoops

HOOP-TO-HOOP HOP

Arrange several hoops in a circle around the room or playground. Have the students form a single row. Read the poem aloud and have the students chant the first verse as they take turns hopping from hoop to hoop:

I hop, hop, hop inside each hoop.
I hop, hop, hop around each loop.

When everyone has had a turn have the students form a double row. Have everyone chant the poem as the partners hop from hoop to hoop:

We hop, hop, hop now two by two.
We hop, hop, hop until we're through.

JUMP THROUGH THE CIRCLE

Have two students hold a hoop several inches from the floor or ground. Tell the other students to form a row and chant the poem aloud as each student takes a turn jumping through the hoop:

Jump through the circle.
Shout, "Hi-dee-hay!"
Now jump through the circle
The other way.

6–29 I'M MARCHING!

Marching is a wonderful way to exercise the whole body.

Materials:

record player or cassette player
record or cassette of lively marching music

Directions:

Have the students line up single file. Play a record or a cassette of marching music. Read the poem aloud and have the students chant it as they march around:

I'm marching, marching,
Marching down the street.
Left foot and right foot
Moving to the beat.

Left foot and right foot
Moving up and down.
I'm marching, marching,
Marching through the town.

6–30 EXERCISE REVIEW SHEETS

This is a good time to review what the children have learned about exercise.

Materials:

copies of review sheets 6–30A through 6–30C
pencils

Directions:

Have copies of these review sheets available. They may be used for review, as independent activities, or they may be placed in learning centers.

Activity Sheets for Section 6: Exercise

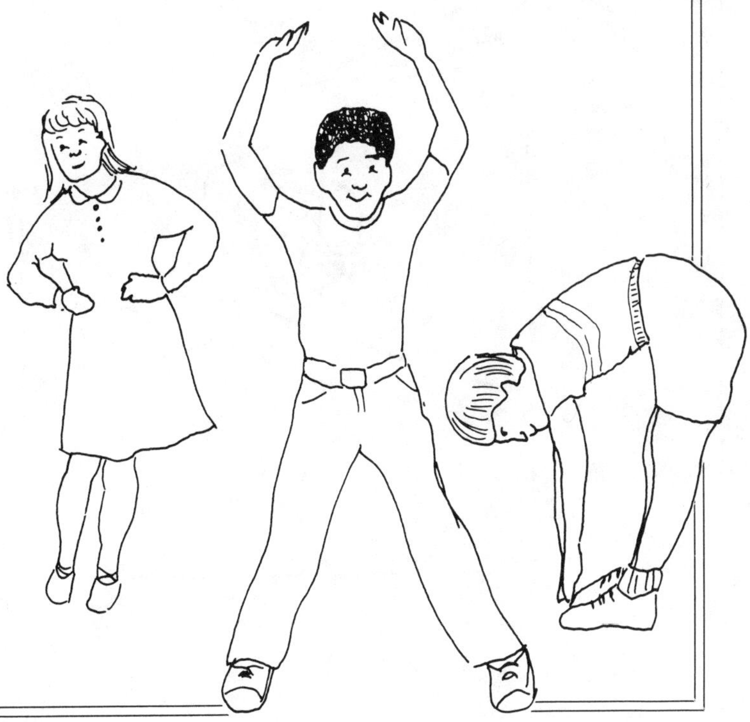

Name ______________________ Date ______________________

FITNESS SIGNS

6–2A

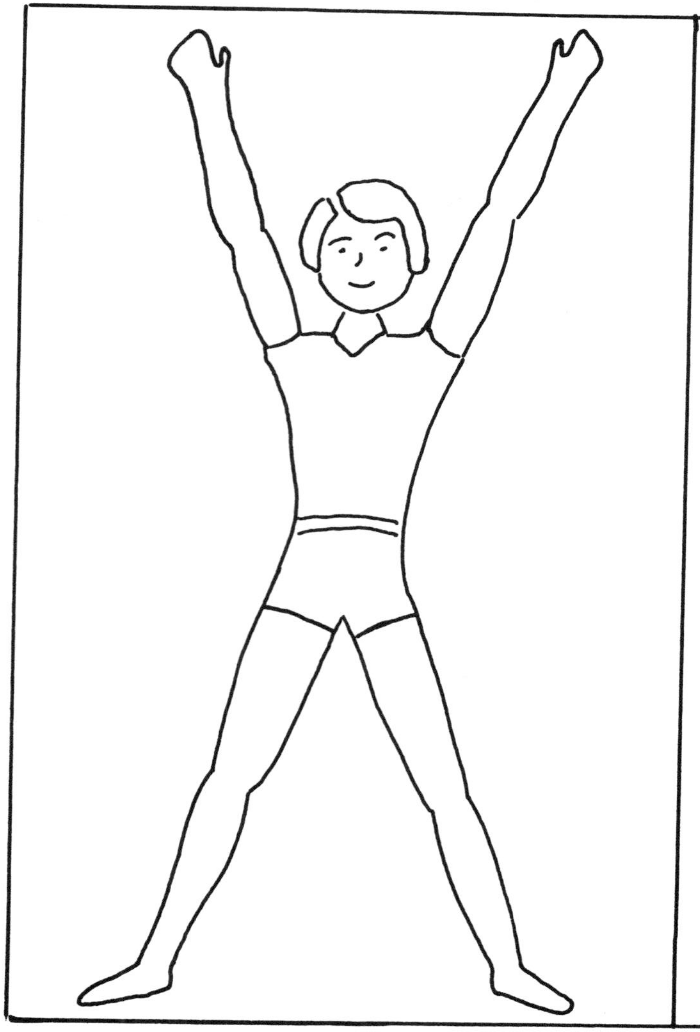

Breathe Deeply

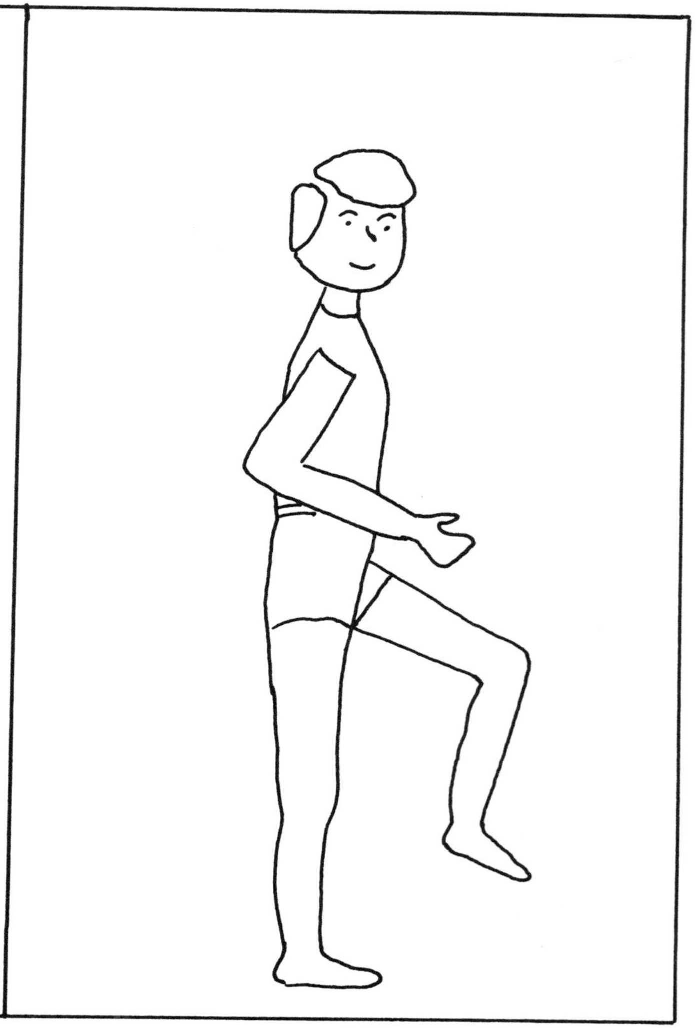

Run in Place

Name ____________________ Date ____________________

FITNESS SIGNS

6–2B

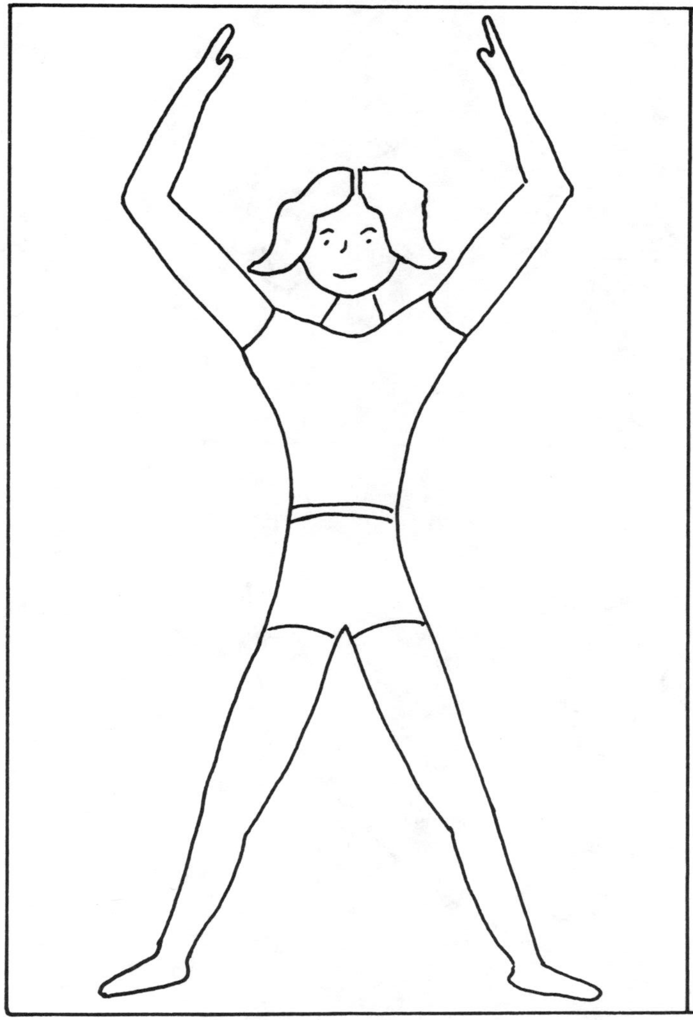

Jumping Jacks

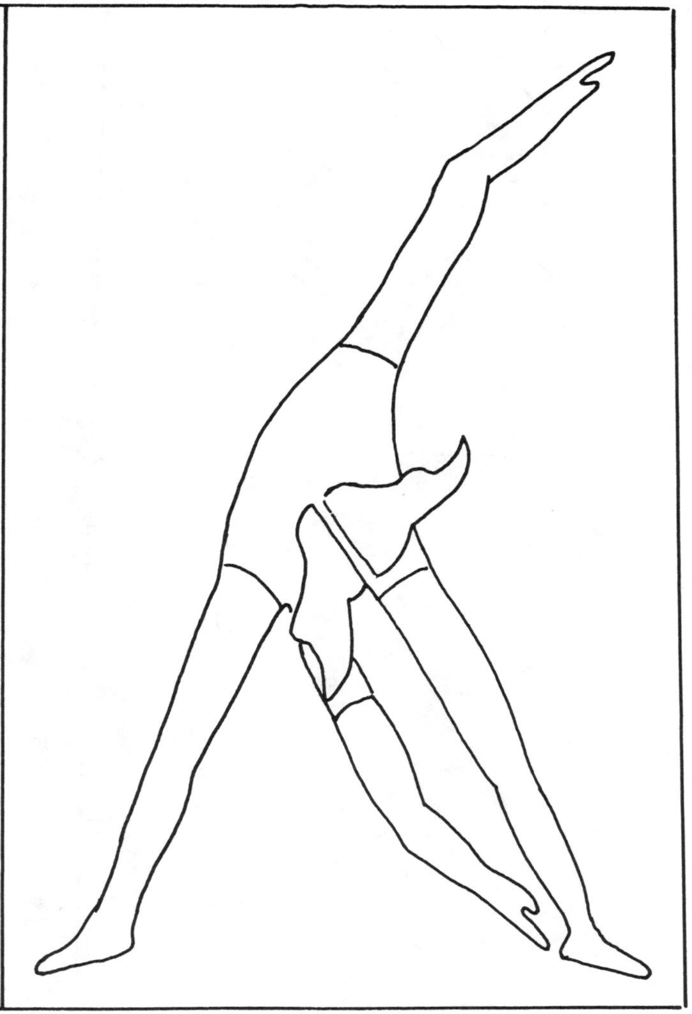

Left Hand/Right Hand Toe Touch

Name ______________________________ Date ________________

EXERCISE WHEEL *6–3A*

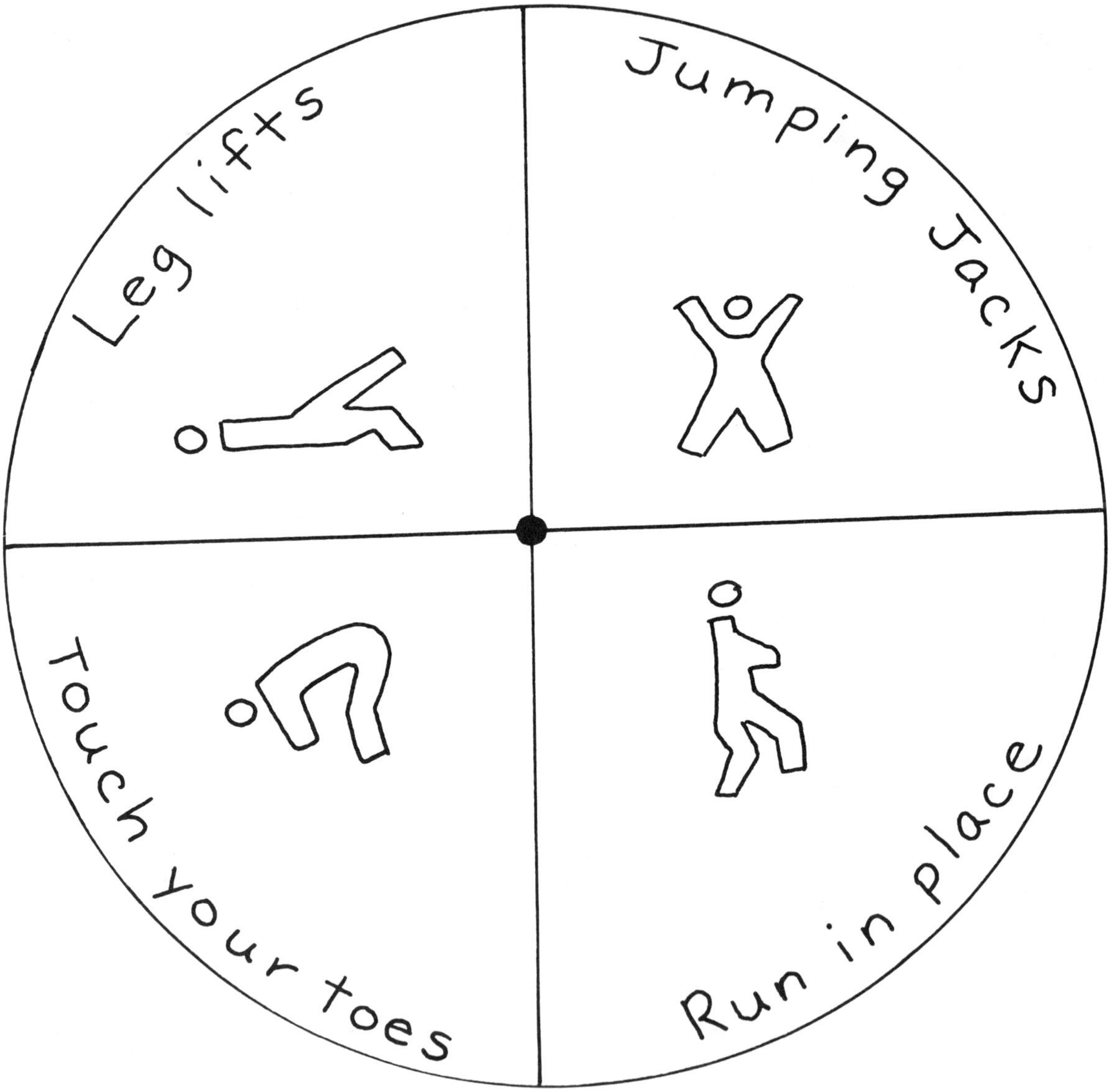

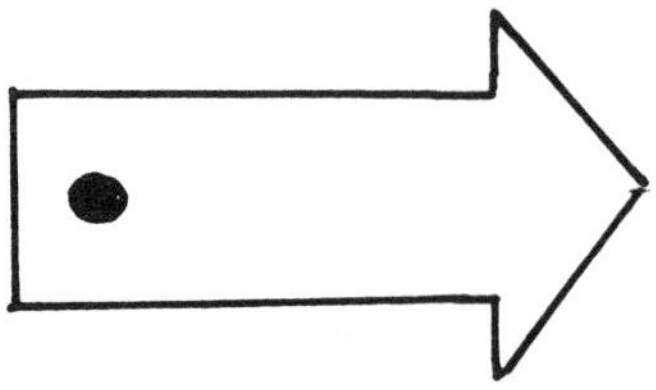

Name ______________________ **Date** ______________________

EXERCISE CHART

6–3B

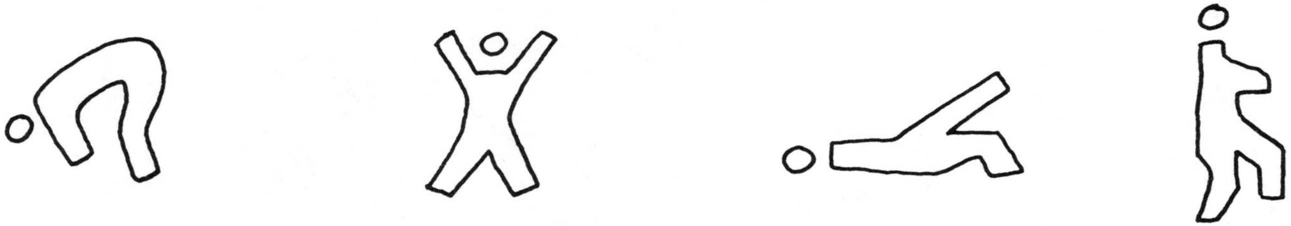

	Mon.	Tues.	Wed.	Thurs.	Fri.	Sat.	Sun.
Week 1							
Week 2							
Week 3							

Exercise every day to stay healthy.

Color a space each time you exercise.

Name ______________________________ Date ____________________

ALPHABET ACTIVITIES *6–30A*

Start at A and connect the dots to see some things to use while you exercise.

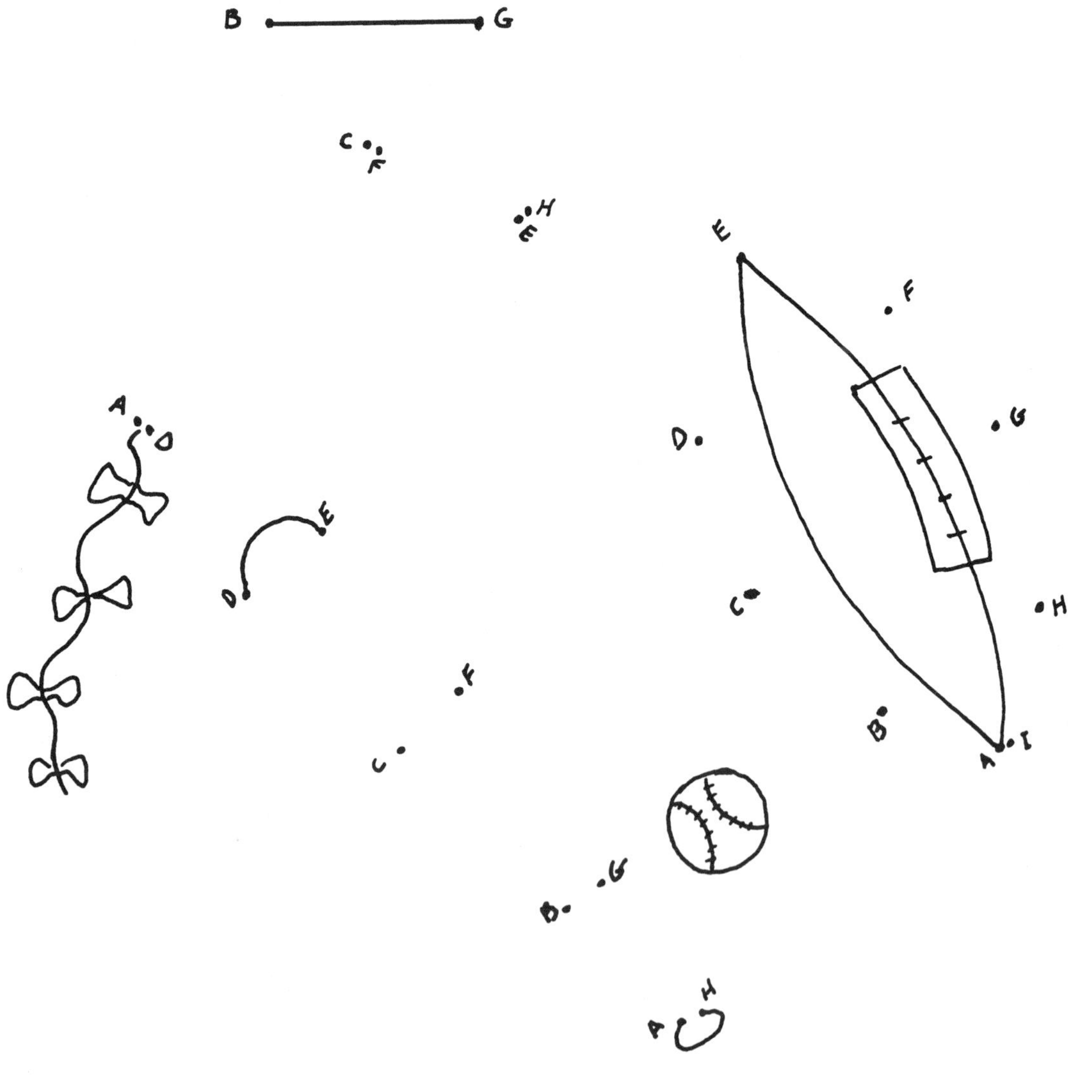

Use some of these dot-to-dot things each day
To make your exercise seem like play.

Name ______________________________ Date ____________________

ALPHABET ACTIVITIES *6–30B*

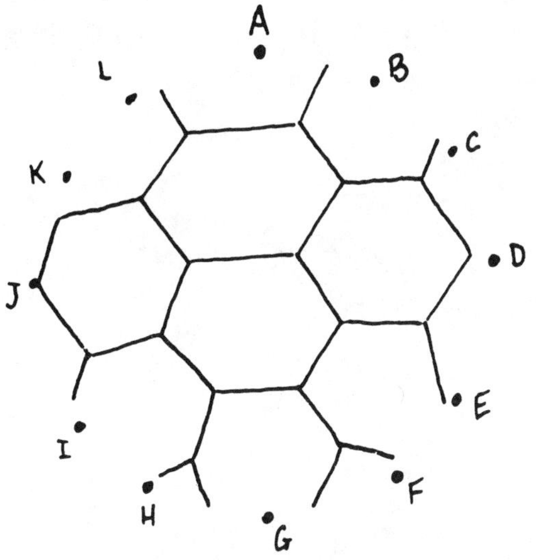

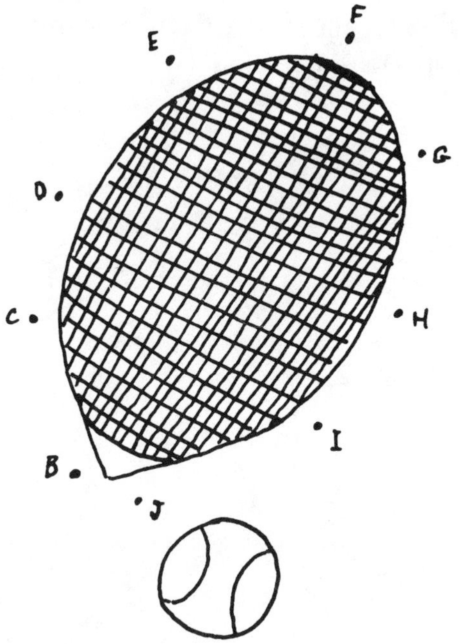

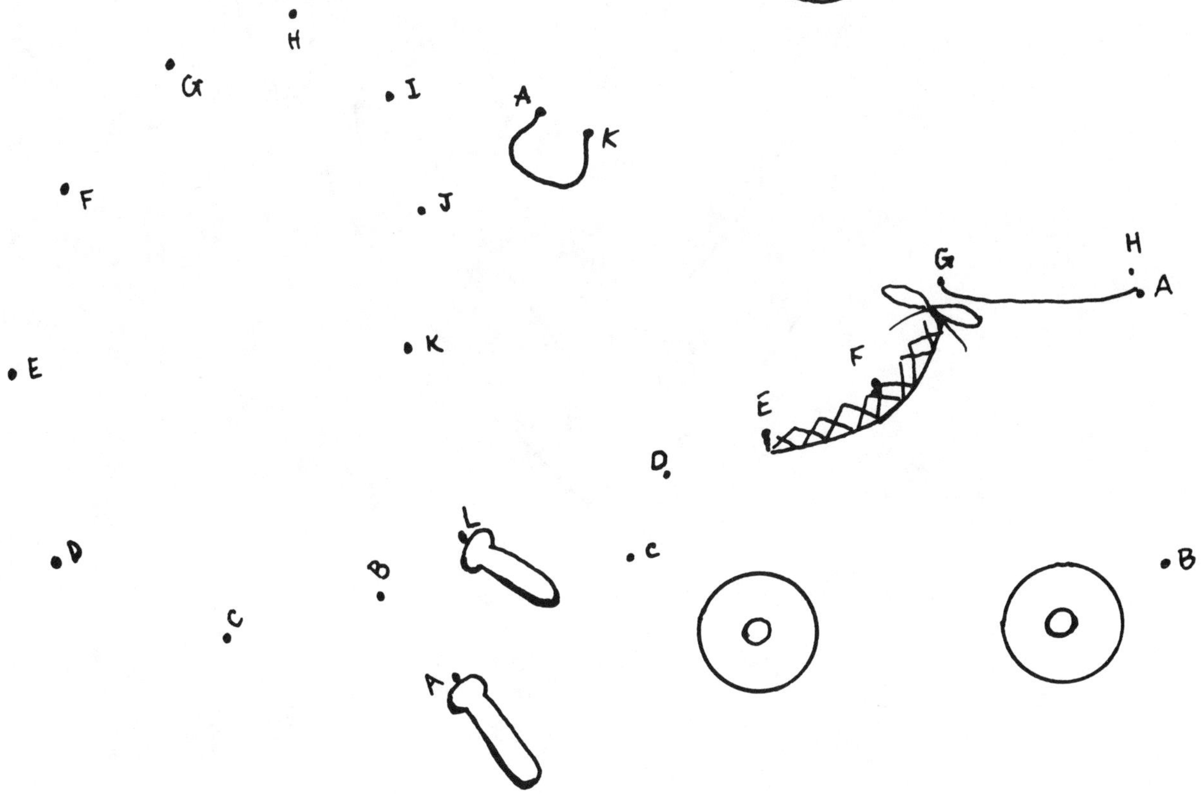

Name ______________________________ Date ________________

HEART HINT *6–30C*

This heart hint will help you keep your heart healthy. Start at the arrow. Circle the first letter and then every other letter until you come to the dot. Write the circled letters in the spaces below the heart.

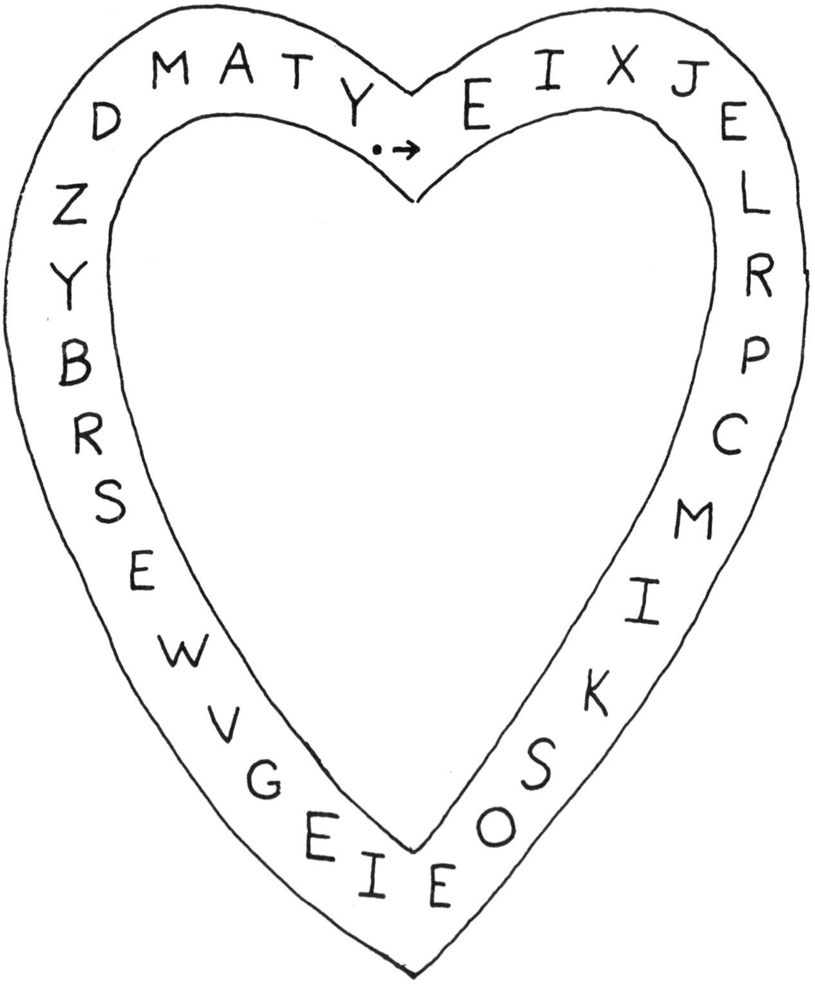

_ _ _ _ _ _ _ _   _ _ _ _ _   _ _ _

7 — SUBSTANCE ABUSE PREVENTION

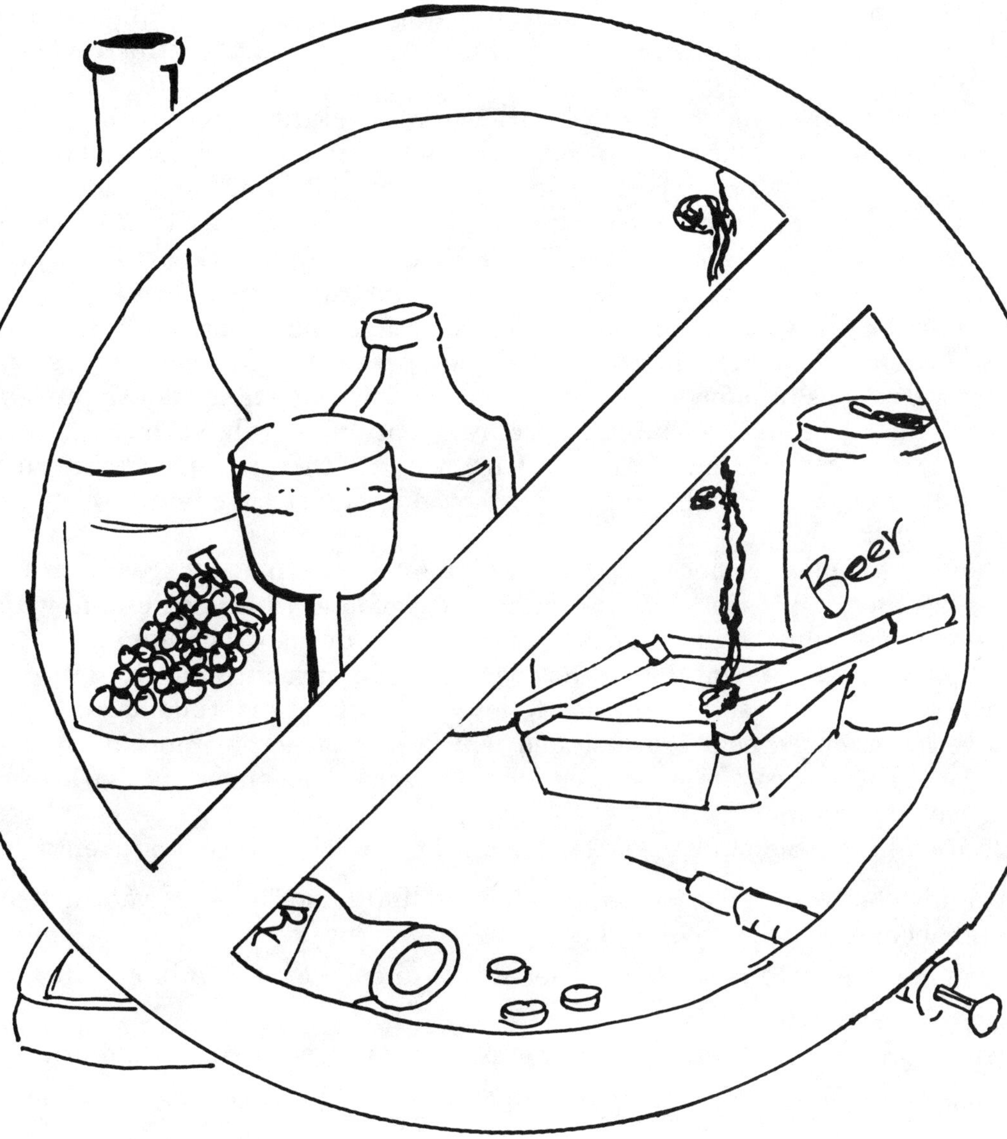

Recent studies among elementary school children found that by the fourth grade, children are already feeling substantial peer pressure to experiment with alcohol and other drugs. Although HAPPY, HEALTHY, AND FIT! is designed to be used with children younger than fourth grade, you can begin now to prepare your students for the pressures they will face in the near future. The attitudes and habits that children learn in their early years can have an important influence on the decisions they make later.

Cigarettes and alcohol are considered "gateway" drugs. Most children who become involved with drugs try them first. Once they become comfortable with cigarettes and alcohol, they may move on to marijuana, amphetamines, cocaine, and other drugs. By teaching children why and how to refuse cigarettes and alcohol, you can reduce their chances of getting involved with any drugs.

Research studies show that helping children develop skills with which to deal with the problems and pressures they face in everyday life is an effective way of helping them resist alcohol and other drugs. Most experts also agree that self-awareness and self-esteem are important factors in children's decisions to try drugs or to refuse them. Refer to the activities in the Feelings and Self-Esteem section of HAPPY, HEALTHY, AND FIT! for ideas on how to help your students become more aware of their own individuality and self-worth.

Current research shows that, to be effective, substance abuse prevention efforts must be reinforced in the home. Look for opportunities during parent-teacher conferences, open houses, and casual conversations to inform students' families about substance abuse prevention activities you are including in the curriculum. Encourage parents to talk with their children about drugs and family values. Children who can talk openly with their parents about drugs are more likely to resist them. The section begins with a reproducible letter to families explaining basic concepts about substance abuse prevention.

Four- to eight-year-olds are not ready for detailed information about specific drugs and their effects. However, they can learn which substances are good for their bodies and which are not; they are able to understand the difference between "good" drugs which help them stay healthy and "bad" drugs which are harmful; and they can learn and practice how to refuse things they know are not healthy. The activities that follow will help your students understand these concepts. Several review sheets are included which reinforce the information presented in earlier activities. These sheets may be used for review, as independent activities, or they may be placed in learning centers.

The activities in the Substance Abuse Prevention section will help students:

- distinguish between "good" drugs which are helpful and "bad" drugs which are harmful to their bodies;
- identify cigarettes, alcohol, and other drugs and become familiar with their general effects on the body;
- develop and practice techniques for refusing cigarettes, alcohol, and other drugs;
- develop problem solving skills which they can apply in everyday situations.

7–1 LETTER TO PARENTS

Date________________________

Dear Parent,

During the next few weeks, your child will be participating in a variety of Substance Abuse Prevention activities. Here are some of the ideas the class will discuss:

- Doctors often prescribe "good" drugs to help people get well when they are sick. Drugs given by parents or doctors are "good" drugs and it is all right to take them.
- Alcohol and cigarettes are "bad" drugs that are harmful to the body.
- Smoking cigarettes hurts the lungs and makes it hard to breathe.
- Drinks that contain alcohol, such as beer or wine, make children feel dizzy and sick. They hurt the brain and make it hard to think clearly.
- Children should always say "NO!" to anyone who wants them to try cigarettes, alcohol, or other "bad" drugs.

Our goals for the Substance Abuse Prevention activities are to help the children recognize substances that are good for their bodies and those that are not, to help them understand the difference between "good" drugs which help them stay healthy and "bad" drugs which are harmful, and to help them develop and practice techniques for refusing substances that they know are not healthy.

In order to be effective, substance abuse prevention efforts must be reinforced in the home. You can help by talking openly with your child about drugs and family values. Take time to listen to your child and show that you respect his or her opinions and concerns. And emphasize the importance of good health by talking about ways people can stay healthy.

Please contact me with any questions you may have about our Substance Abuse Prevention activities.

Sincerely,

____

Your child's teacher

7–2 SUBSTANCE ABUSE DISCUSSION

Many children are exposed to alcohol, cigarettes, and drugs as early as the fourth grade. Help your students learn why these substances are harmful and how to resist pressure to try them.

Materials:

copies of Substance Abuse Pictures page 7–2A
copies of Yes/No page 7–2B
scissors
glue
index cards or 3″ construction paper squares
old magazines
9″ x 12″ construction paper

Preparation:

1. Cut apart one Substance Abuse Pictures page to make 12 individual pictures.
2. Glue each small picture to an index card or a construction paper square.
3. Cut out cigarette and alcohol ads from old magazines. Glue the magazine ads to construction paper and display on a bulletin board.

Directions:

Begin by asking students what they know about drugs. Encourage an open discussion; listen to the children's ideas and experiences but refrain from making judgmental comments. Then discuss the following concepts with students. As you discuss each harmful substance, point out a picture of it on the bulletin board.

- Doctors often prescribe "good" drugs that help people get well when they are sick. Drugs your parents or doctor gives you are "good" drugs and it is all right to take them.
- Alcohol and cigarettes are "bad" drugs that hurt our bodies.
- Smoking cigarettes hurts our lungs and makes it hard to breathe.
- Drinks that contain alcohol, such as beer or wine, make children feel dizzy and sick. They hurt the brain and make it hard to think clearly.
- Children who try alcohol or cigarettes often use other "bad" drugs later.
- You should always say "NO!" to anyone who wants you to try alcohol, cigarettes, or other "bad" drugs.

After the discussion, distribute the Substance Abuse Pictures pages. Have students make picture cards, following the directions in "Preparation."

Work with a small group and have students spread their picture cards face up on their desks. Hold up your set of pictures, one by one, and ask students to find the matching pictures. Have students tell which things are all right to use and which are not. Remind them that the pills and the syringe are all right if they are given by a parent or a doctor. Stress that children should never take pills or other medicines they find around the house.

Distribute the Yes/No pages and have students read the tags on the containers. Then ask students to classify their Substance Abuse picture cards by laying pictures of things that are all right on the container marked "Yes" and those that are harmful on the container marked "No." If some students put the bottle of pills and the syringe on the "Yes" container, ask them to explain their reasons.

7–3 SUBSTANCE ABUSE GAME

Use this game to help children learn to distinguish between substances that are harmful and those that are not.

Materials:

copies of Substance Abuse Game Sheet 7–3A
a button for each student
one die for every three or four students

Directions:

Divide students into groups of three or four and let each student choose a button to use as a game marker. Give each group a Substance Abuse Game Sheet and a die.

Point out the START space on the game sheet, and have students place their game markers there. Explain that the players in each group will take turns tossing the die and moving their buttons the number of spaces shown. When they land on a space with a picture, they should name the picture, tell whether or not it is something that is all right to use, and explain why or why not. Read aloud the words that appear on three of the spaces, and explain what players should do if their markers land on those spaces. Encourage each group to continue playing the game until all members of the group reach the FINISH line.

Afterwards, give each of the students a Substance Abuse Game Sheet to add to their "Here's to My Health" booklet file folders. Encourage them to play the game at home with their families and friends.

7–4 REFUSING DRUGS

Children who have practiced saying "No" to drugs find it easier to resist when they are offered drugs. Provide opportunities for your students to practice ways to refuse harmful substances.

Materials:

Substance Abuse Pictures 7–2A, cut apart

role-playing props such as plastic glasses, empty soda bottles, empty pill containers, and others

copies of What Will You Say? activity sheet 7–4A

Directions:

Help students recall which substances are harmful and which are not by shuffling one set of Substance Abuse Pictures and holding them up, one by one. Tell students to clap and shout HOORAY! when they see a picture of something that is all right to eat or drink, and to stamp their feet and shout BOO! for pictures of things that hurt the body and should not be used.

Lead a discussion of what students might say and do if others want them to try things they know will hurt their bodies. Write these sentences on the chalkboard:

- No, smoke makes me cough.
- No, I promised my parents that I wouldn't use drugs.
- No, I want to be healthy.

Encourage students to think of other things to say, and add their ideas to the list. Discuss other ways of refusing drugs, such as walking away from the person who is offering them, ignoring the person, staying away from people they know use drugs, or changing the subject and talking about something else.

Help students practice ways to refuse drugs by having them role play how they would act and what they would say if someone offered them drugs. Divide students into groups of two or three and ask each group to plan a short skit in which one student pretends to offer drugs to one or two others who refuse them. Point out the props that are available for students to use if they wish. Move around the room while the groups are planning their skits and give help, if needed. Remind students to refer to the list on the chalkboard of ways to refuse drugs.

After a few minutes, have groups take turns presenting their skits for the class. When all the groups have presented their skits, distribute the What Will You Say? activity sheets. Read the directions on the page aloud with students, and then help them write what they would say and do if someone offered them drugs. Again, refer them to the list on the chalkboard if they need help thinking of ways to refuse drugs.

7–5 SUBSTANCE ABUSE ACTIVITIES

Using a game format can be an effective way of having students practice ways to refuse drugs. Ask students to find partners for the following activities. Give each pair a set of Substance Abuse picture cards (see activity 7–2).

SOMETHING FOR YOU

Have pairs of students thoroughly shuffle one set of Substance Abuse picture cards and place them face down in a pile. Tell students to take turns drawing the top card and showing it to their partners as they chant this verse:

Hello! Hello!
How do you do?
Here is something
I have for you.

When the second student has seen the picture on the card, he or she must respond by verbally accepting or refusing it. In either case, the student should give reasons for the acceptance or refusal. For example, the student might say, "Thank you, I love ice cream!" or "No, I don't want to hurt my body by smoking." Have students continue until they have drawn all the cards in the pile.

DO YOU REMEMBER?

Tell one student in each pair to lay four to six Substance Abuse picture cards face up on the table in front of their partners. Tell the partners to look carefully at the pictures and try to remember what they are. After a few seconds, they should close their eyes while the one who put the cards out removes one or two cards. The partners then open their eyes and try to name the cards that are missing. If the missing cards show things that are all right to eat or drink, the students should ask for them back and tell why they want them. If they are things that should not be used, the students should tell what they would say if someone offered those things to them. Then have students switch roles and repeat the game.

7–6 PROBLEM-SOLVING SKILLS

Research shows that children who know how to cope with pressures and problems are more likely to resist peer pressure to try drugs. Practicing problem solving skills will prepare your students to handle everyday situations without resorting to drugs.

Ask students to tell about problems they encounter at school, at home, or in their neighborhoods. For example: A classmate is having a birthday party but didn't invite you; your best friend says he doesn't like you and won't play with you anymore; your mom is angry and punishes you because you forgot to feed the dog.

As students describe each problem, write a brief description of it on the chalkboard. When the list is complete, circle several of the most common problems. Then ask students to help brainstorm ways to handle those situations.

Explain that, in brainstorming, any idea is acceptable. Read aloud the description of one of the problems. Then make a separate list of all the ways students mention to solve or handle that problem. Compliment the class for thinking of so many ways to solve the problem, and then reread the list of solutions aloud. Ask students to decide which are the best ways to handle the problem. There will probably be some disagreement about the best way to handle the problem. Emphasize that different people react to situations in different ways, and that there is always more than one way to solve a problem.

Continue to brainstorm ways to handle other problems on the list. You may wish to have students role play some of the problems and their solutions.

7–7 SUBSTANCE ABUSE PREVENTION REVIEW SHEETS

This is a good time to review what the children have learned about substance abuse prevention.

Materials:

copies of review sheets 7–7A through 7–7F
pencils

Directions:

Have copies of these review sheets available. They may be used for review, as independent activities, or they may be placed in learning centers.

Activity Sheets for Section 7: Substance Abuse Prevention

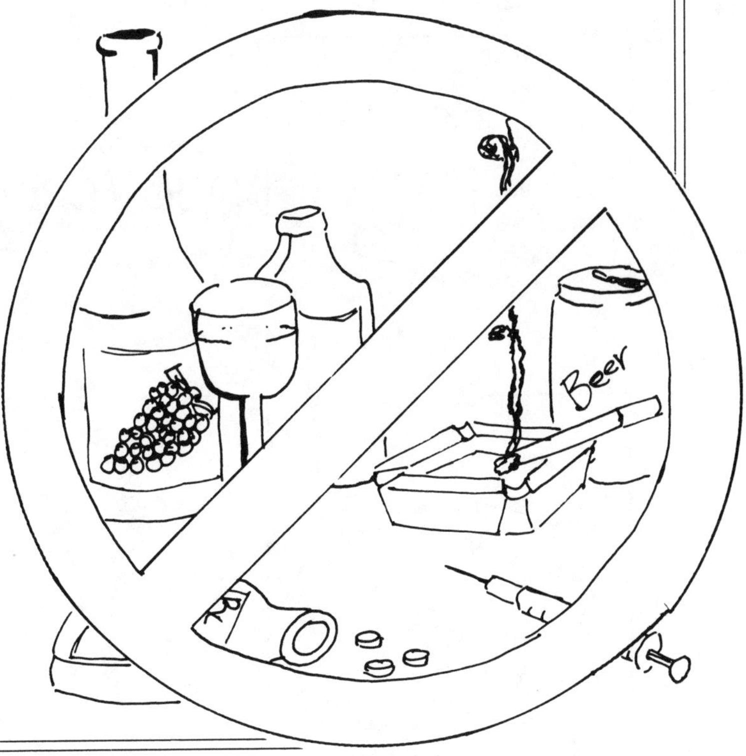

Name ______________________________ Date ________________

SUBSTANCE ABUSE PICTURES *7–2A*

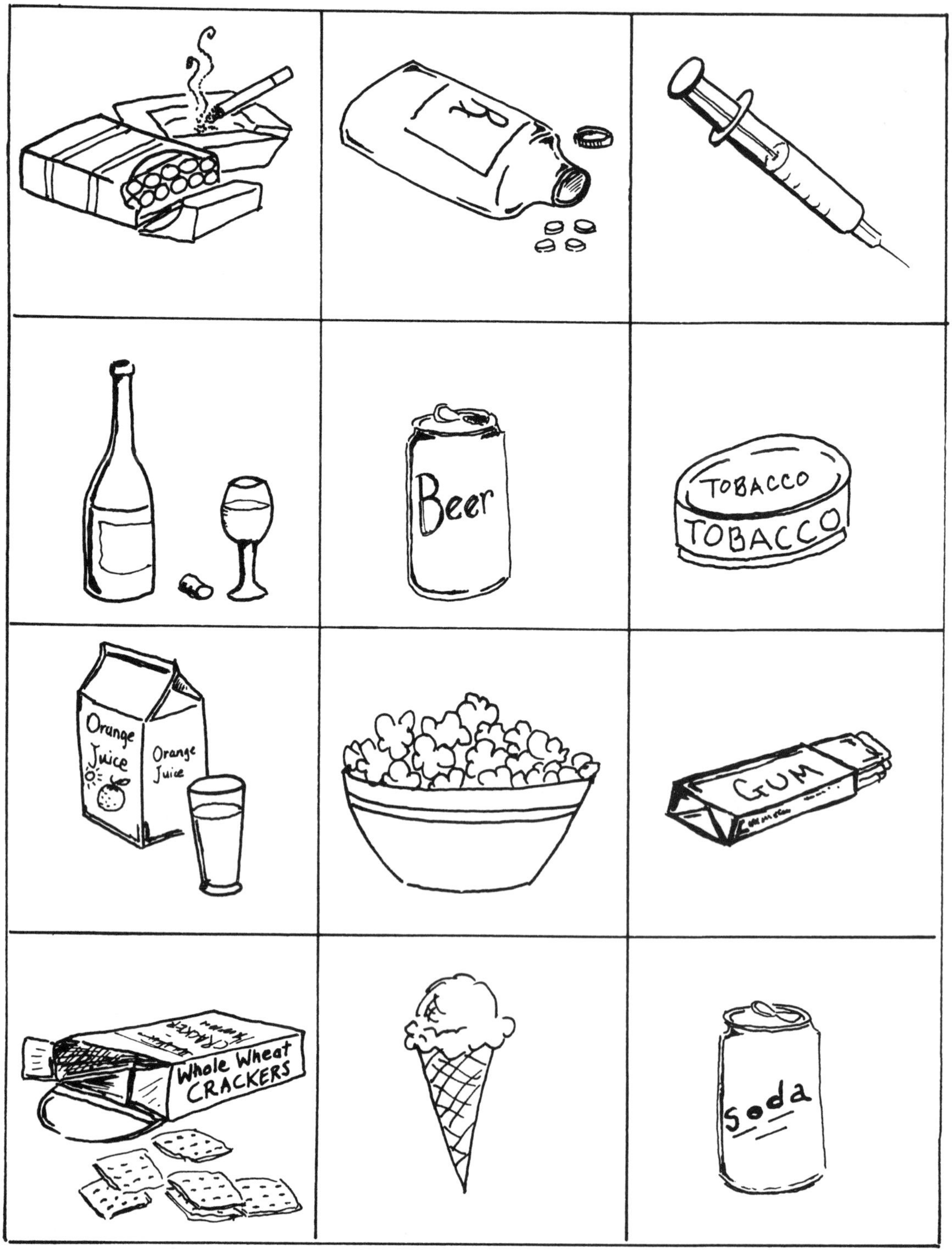

Name ______________________________ Date ______________

YES/NO

7–2B

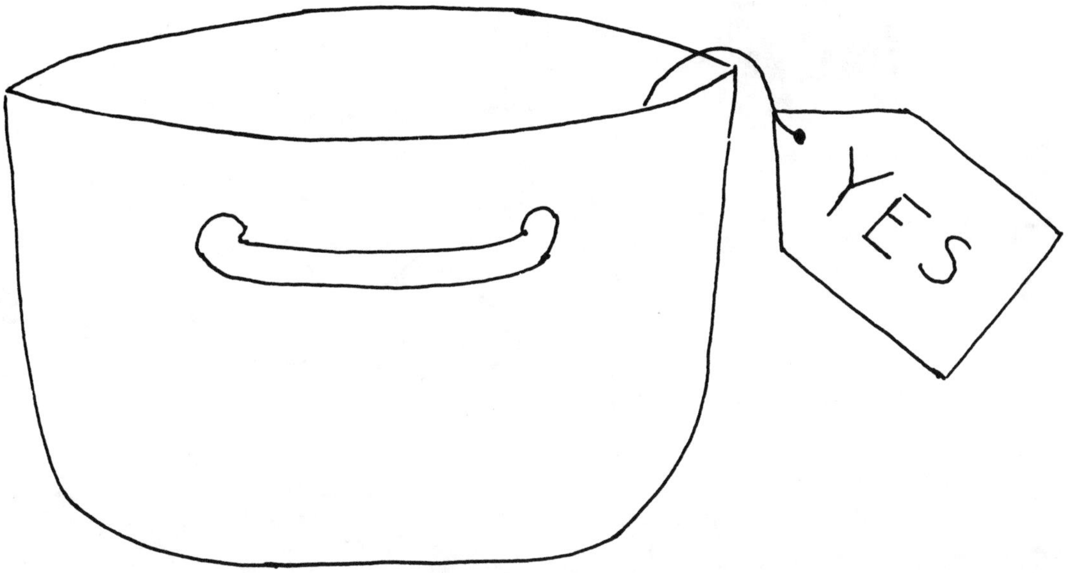

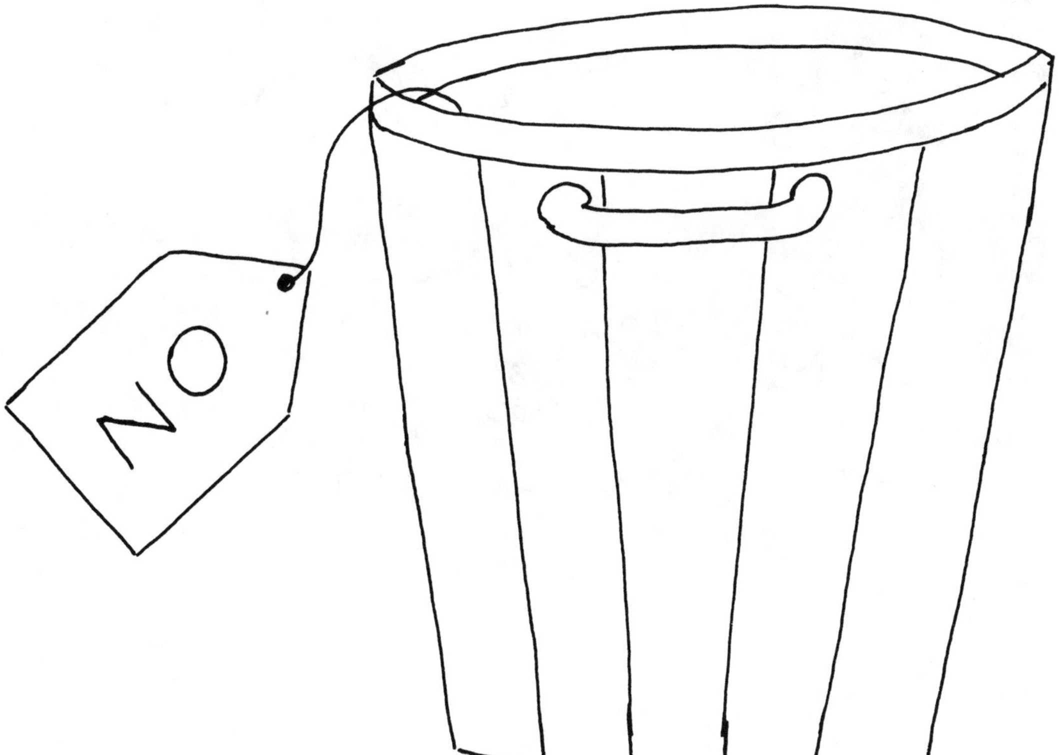

Name ______________________ Date ______________________

SUBSTANCE ABUSE GAME SHEET 7–3A

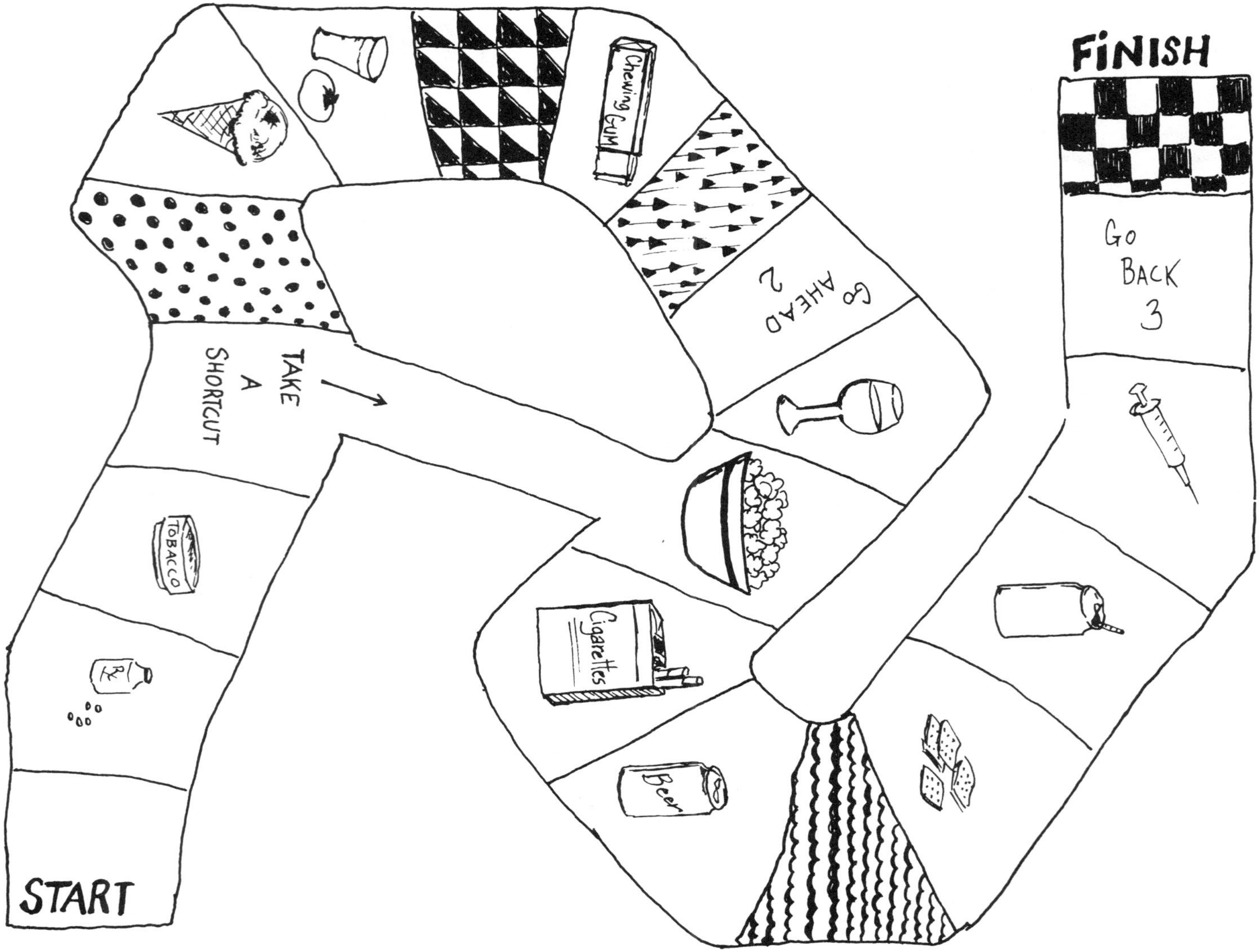

Name ______________________________ Date ________________

WHAT WILL YOU SAY? *7–4A*

These are things you should never use. They hurt your body. They keep you from being healthy.

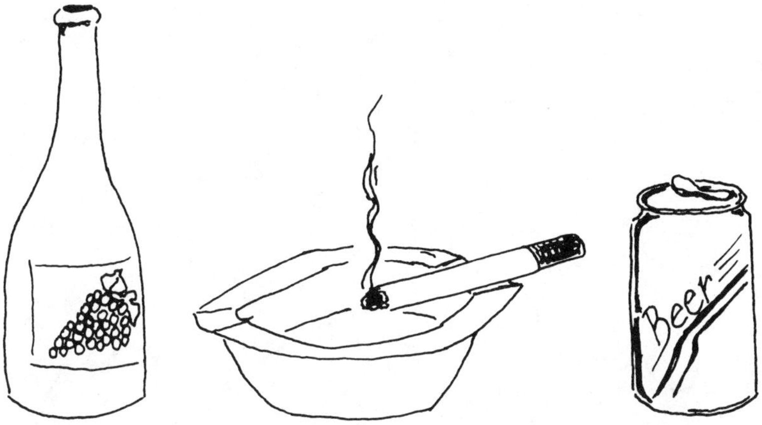

What will you say if someone wants you to try them?

____

____

What will you do if the person keeps asking you to try them?

____

____

Name ______________________________ Date ________________

DRUG WARNING

7–7A

To solve this drug warning puzzle, start at the arrow. Circle the first letter and then every other letter until you come to the exclamation points. Write the circled letters below.

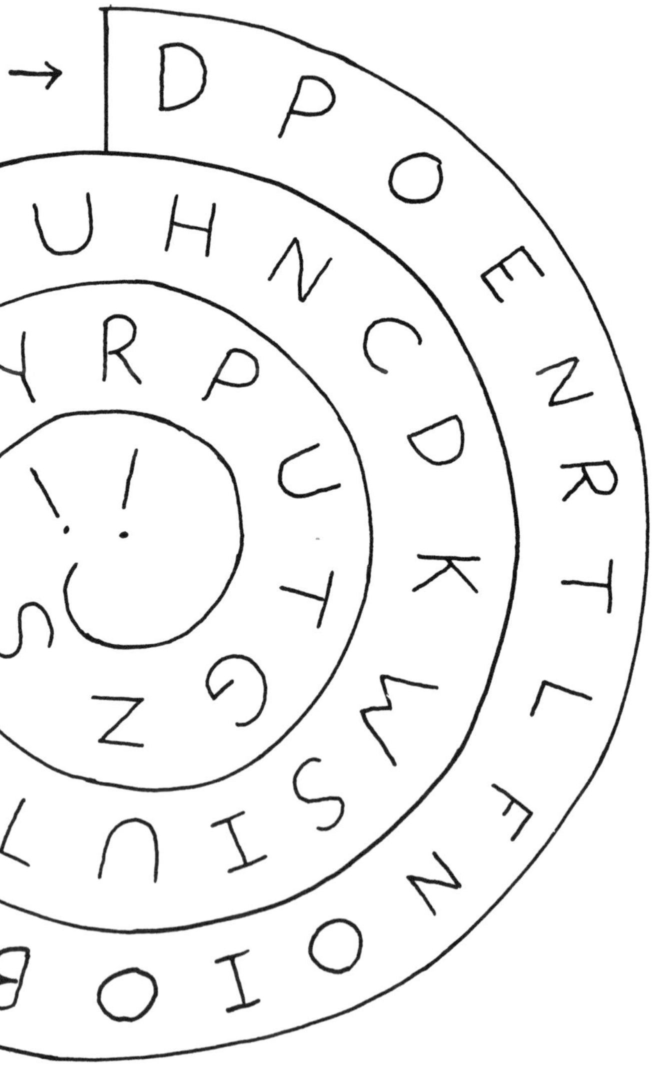

_ _ _ _   _ _ _ _ _ _   _ _ _ _ _ _ _

_ _ _ _   _ _ _ _ _ _ !!

Name ______________________________ **Date** ______________

BE SAFE *7–7B*

Many things around the house can make you sick if you put them in your mouth. Do not eat or drink anything unless you are sure it is safe.

Color the things on the table that are safe to eat or drink. Put an X on the ones that can hurt you.

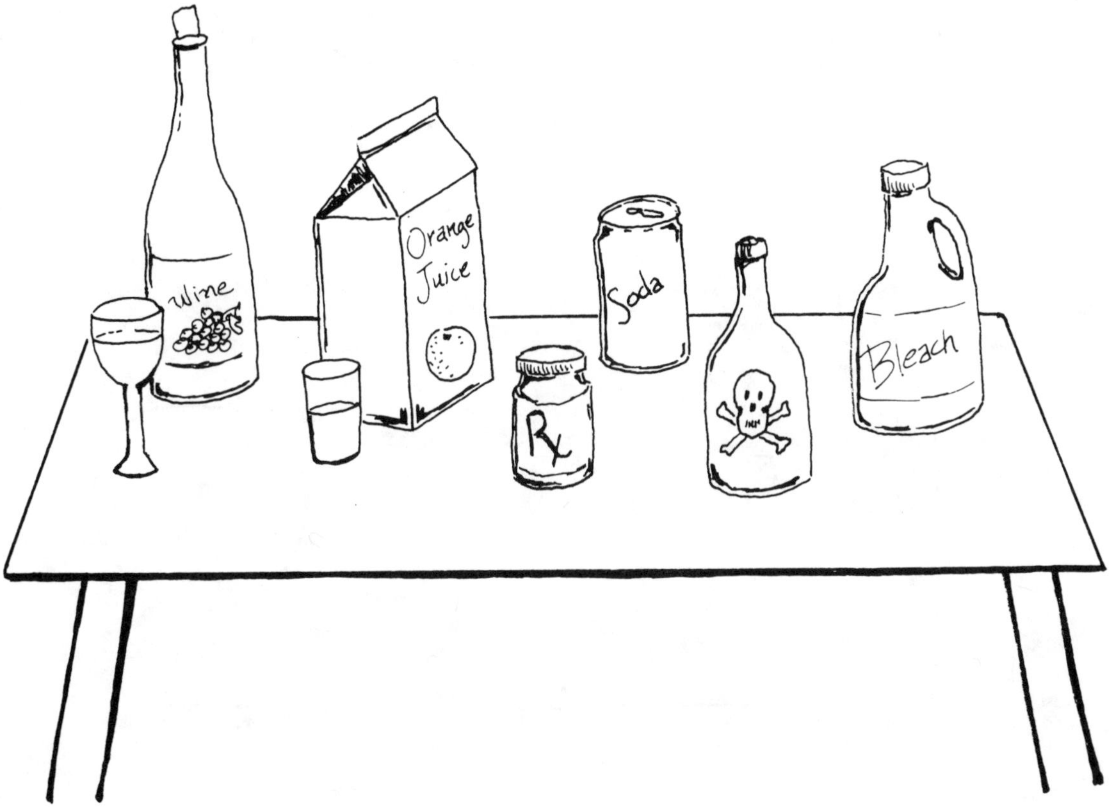

Name ______________________ Date ______________

JUST SAY NO *7–7C*

Begin at the star and connect the dots to find out what to say if someone wants you to try something you know will hurt your body.

Color the letters bright red to help you remember the word.

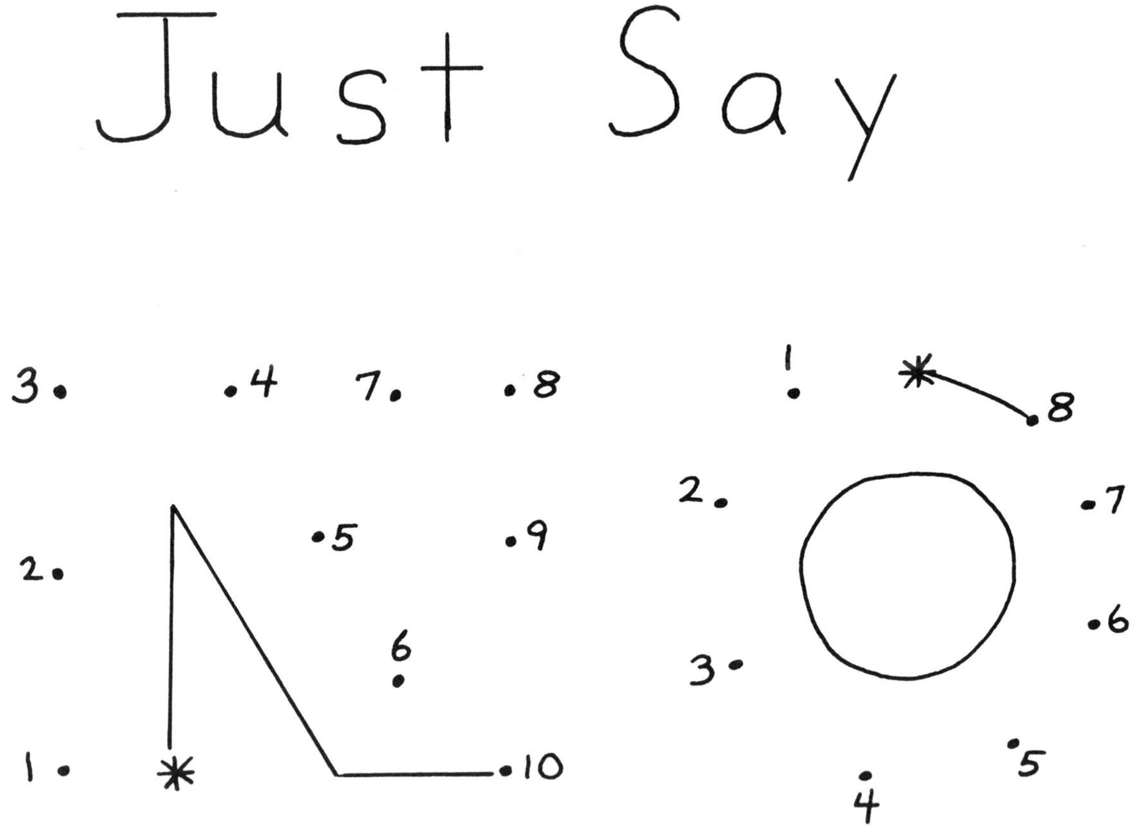

Name ______________________ Date ______________

SUBSTANCE ABUSE MESSAGE *7–7D*

Color the spaces with the dots to find out the warning about drugs.

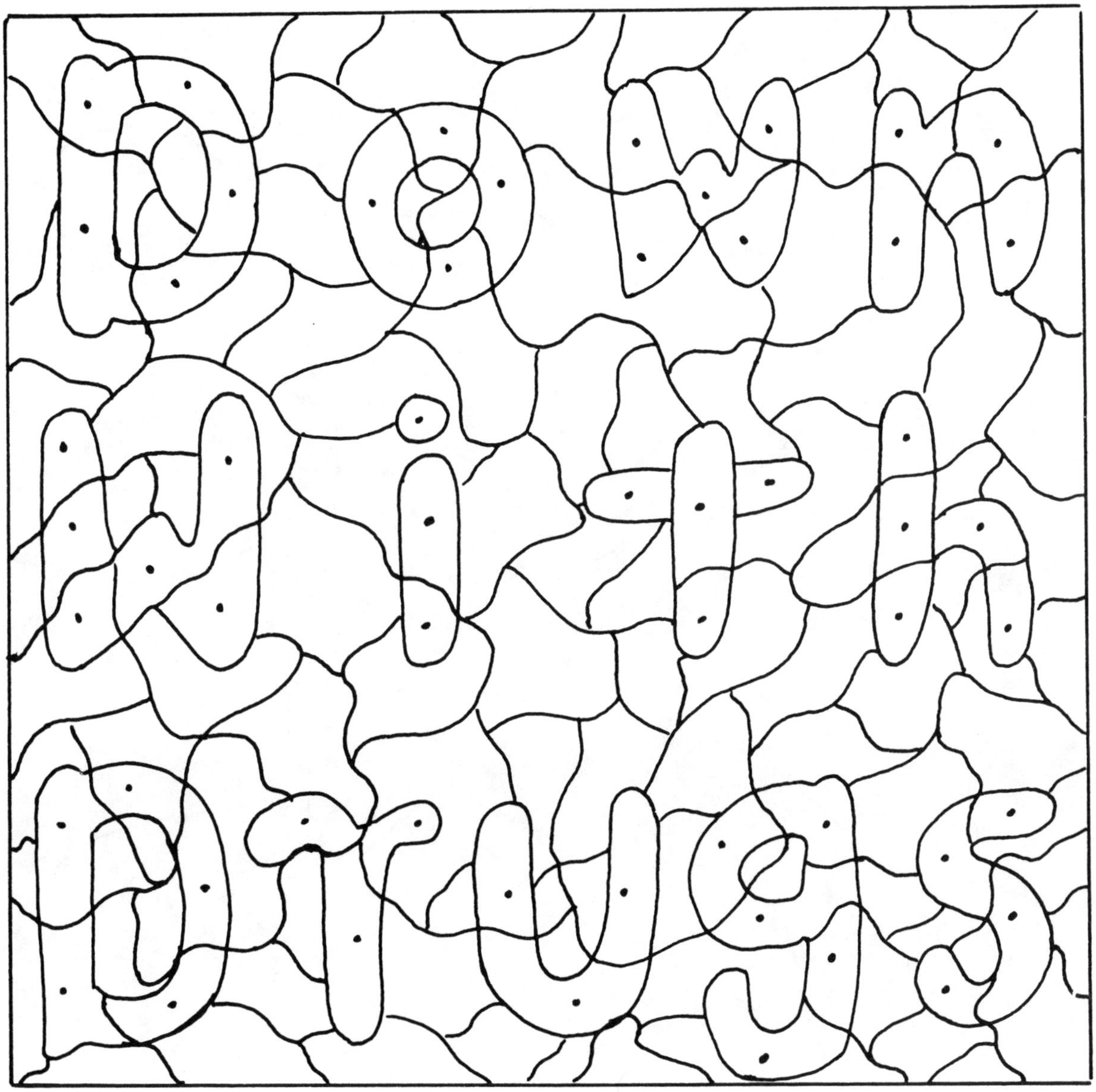

Name ______________________________ Date ________________

DRUG DANGER *7–7E*

To find the hidden warning, start at the arrow. Circle the first letter and then every other letter until you come to the exclamation point. Write the circled letters below.

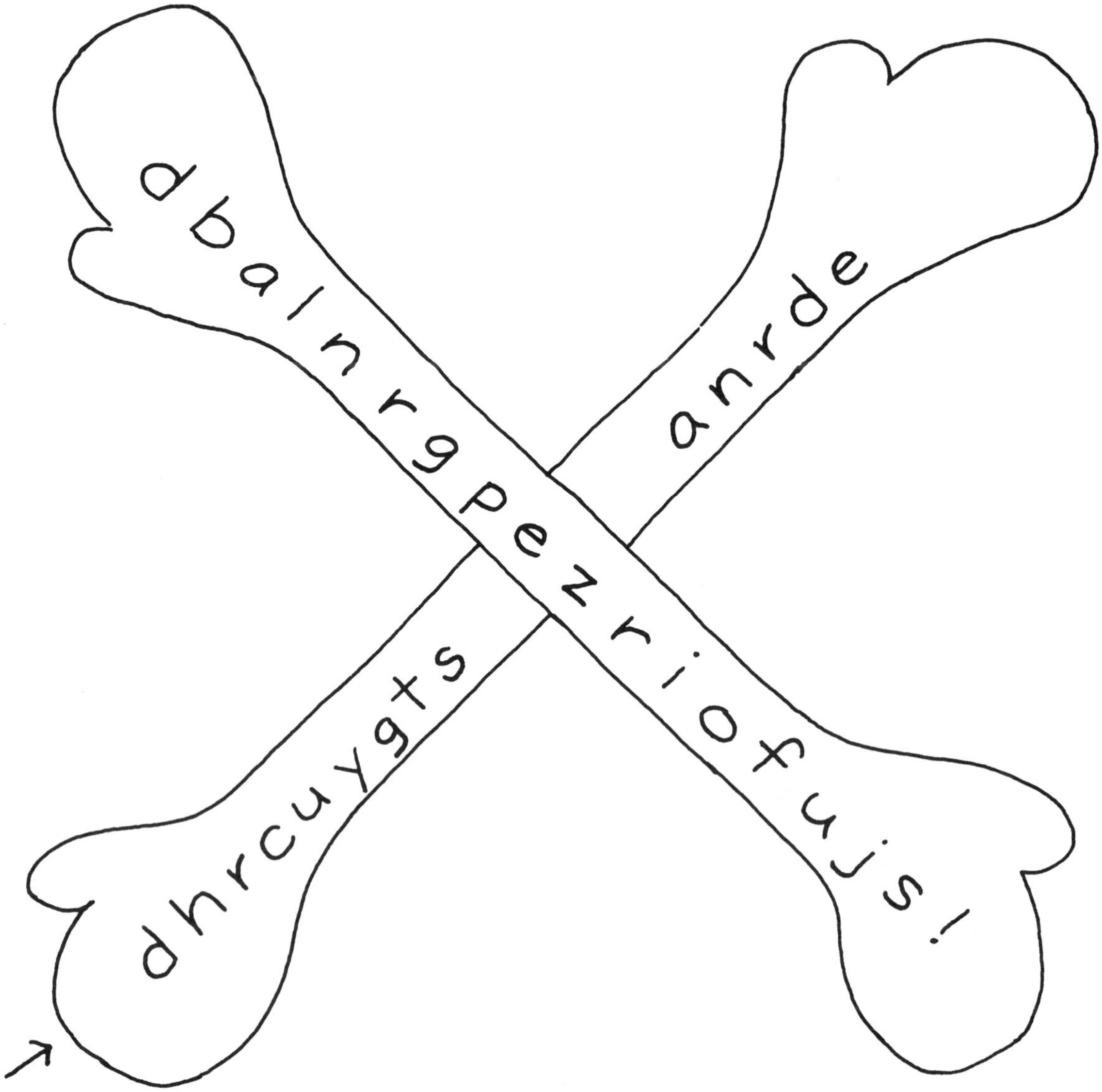

_ _ _ _ _ _ _ _ _ _ _ _ _ _ _ _ _ _ !

Name ______________________ Date ______________

PICK-A-PATH *7–7F*

Put your finger on the X. Move your finger along the path until you come to something that is good for you to eat and drink. Do not cross any lines. Then try it again with a pencil or crayon. Put an X on each thing that will hurt your body.

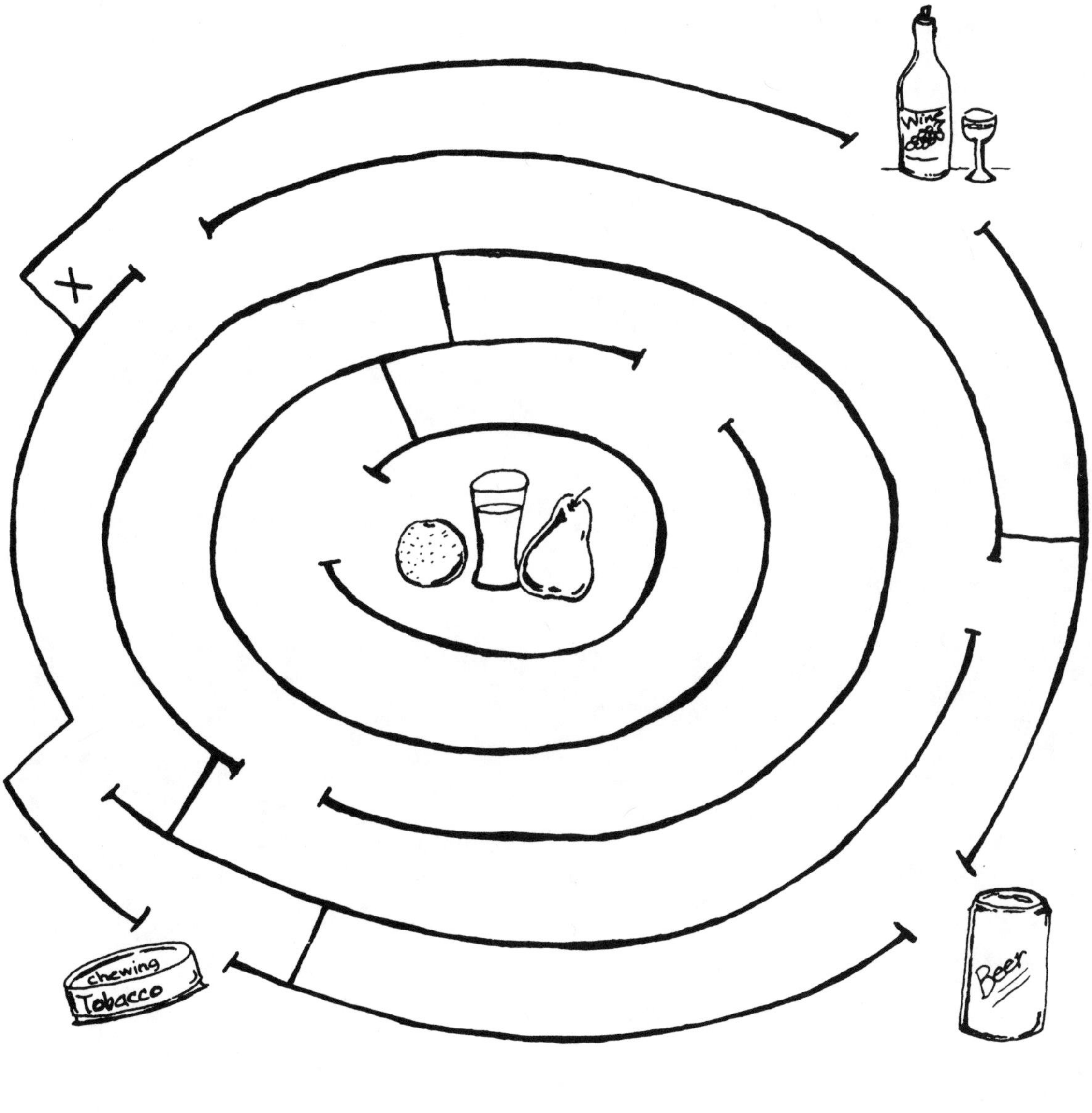

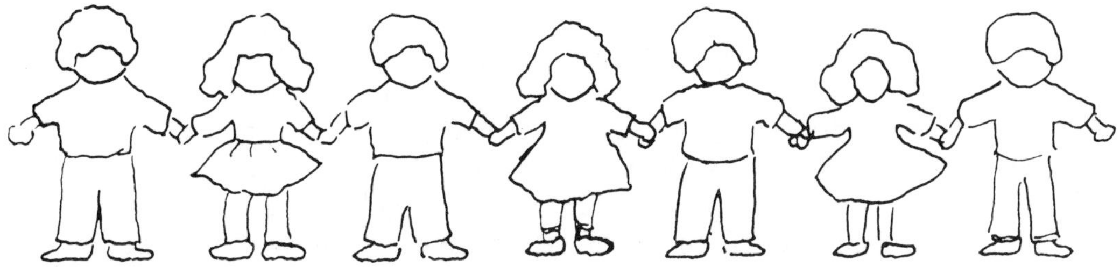

8 = *GAMES AND DANCES*

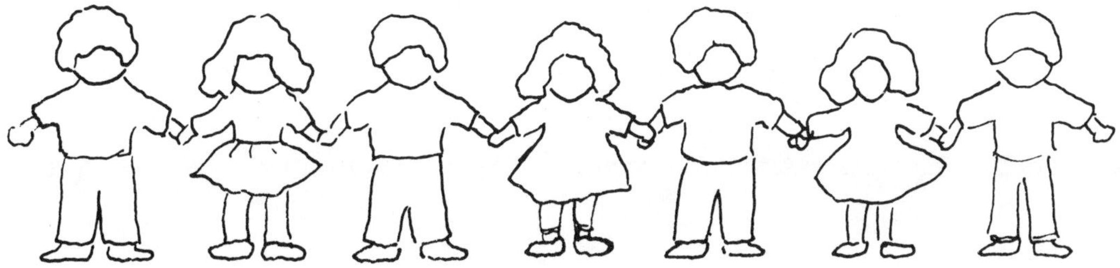

Young children enjoy playing games. Games give them opportunities to interact and socialize with one another as well as to move and exercise their growing bodies and muscles. Games also promote cooperation, help students develop listening skills, and give them practice in following directions.

The games in HAPPY, HEALTHY, AND FIT! are noncompetitive. The object of the games is not for one person or team to win but for all students to participate and have fun. Discourage students from focusing on winning and losing; suggest instead that they each try to improve their own skills and performance.

Dancing and creative movement can also be important forms of exercise. They help students develop balance, body awareness, and muscle control. Through bending, stretching, swaying, and other movements, students improve their posture and learn to move gracefully and easily. You may wish to beat a drum or shake a tambourine to accompany the dances and set the tempo for some of the creative movement activities.

Many of the games and dances in this section supplement and reinforce concepts introduced in other sections of HAPPY, HEALTHY, AND FIT! Use the games and dances to enrich lesson planning, when shifting from one activity to another, or when you have spare minutes during the day.

If some students in your class prefer not to participate in the games and dances, encourage them but don't force them. They may need to observe for a while until they feel confident about what is happening and understand what is expected of them. It may help if you stand nearby and encourage reluctant students to sway or clap while the rest of the class participates in the activity.

The activities in the Games and Dances section will help students:

- interact with one another in structured and unstructured situations;
- exercise large and small muscles;
- develop balance, body awareness, and muscle control;
- have opportunities to be both a leader and a follower in a variety of activities;
- learn to listen and follow directions;
- work together cooperatively to accomplish a common goal.

8–1 SHARK!

Materials:

two old sheets or blankets

Directions:

Put two old sheets on the floor a few feet apart. Assign one player to be the shark. The other players are swimmers. Tell the swimmers to swim around the two islands (sheets). Have the shark swim in and out among the swimmers. At any time you call out, "SHARK!", the swimmers must try to swim to an island and stand on it before the shark tags them. The shark tries to lightly tag as many swimmers as he can. Any swimmers tagged while they are in the ocean become sharks.

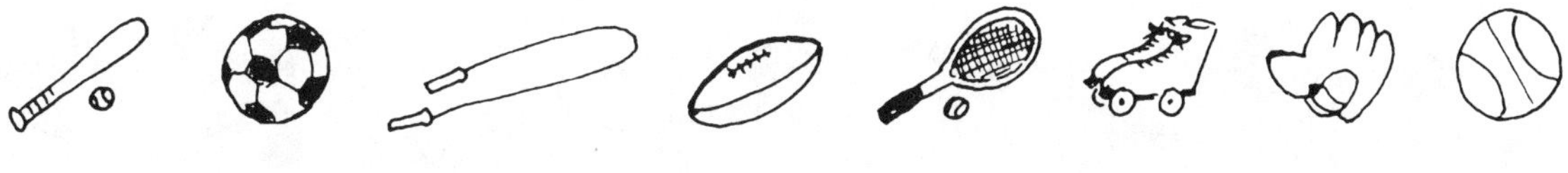

8–2 FIVE GIANT JUMPS

Materials:

string

small markers for each player

Directions:

Put a long piece of string on the playground. Have the players line up single file along the string. Tell them to listen for your clap then the first player in the line counts to five and jumps five giant jumps. Put a small marker at his or her landing place. Have the others see how far they can jump. When everyone has had a turn begin the game again. Ask the players if they can jump a longer distance. Vary the game by having the players jump with a partner.

8–3 PAPER PLATE PEANUT PUSH

Materials:

small paper plates
peanuts

Directions:

Chalk a long starting line on the floor or playground. Chalk a parallel line about 15 feet away. Have the players line up along one line. Give every player a small paper plate. Put a peanut down in front of each player. Tell them to listen for your clap, then bend over and push their peanuts with the paper plates across the finish line. When every player has crossed the finish line have them turn around and push their peanuts back to the starting line.

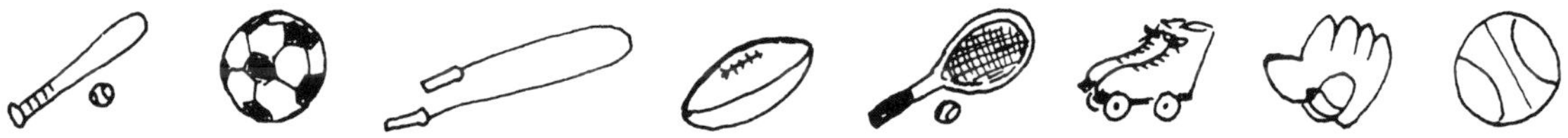

8–4 RED LIGHT!

Materials:

string

Directions:

Lay a piece of string on the playground. Put another piece of string parallel to it about 25 feet away. Assign one player to be IT. Have the other players line up behind a starting line. Tell IT to stand halfway between the two lines with his or her back to the other players. Have IT close his or her eyes and slowly count to ten aloud. While IT is counting the other players must run quickly towards the finish line. Whenever IT calls out, "Red light!", the other players must stop and stand like statues. If IT sees anyone move, that person must return to the starting line. IT begins counting to ten again and the other players continue moving towards the finish line. Continue until everyone has crossed the finish line.

8–5 STOP AND GO GALLOP

Materials:

string
green scarf
red scarf

Directions:

Lay a piece of string on the playground. Put another piece of string parallel to it about 25 feet away. Have the players line up along the starting line. Assign one player to be the traffic officer. Give the traffic officer a green scarf and a red scarf. Ask the traffic officer to stand halfway between the two lines. When the traffic officer holds up the green scarf the players must gallop towards the finish line. When the traffic officer holds up the red scarf the players must stop. Continue until everyone has crossed the finish line and has had a turn being the traffic officer.

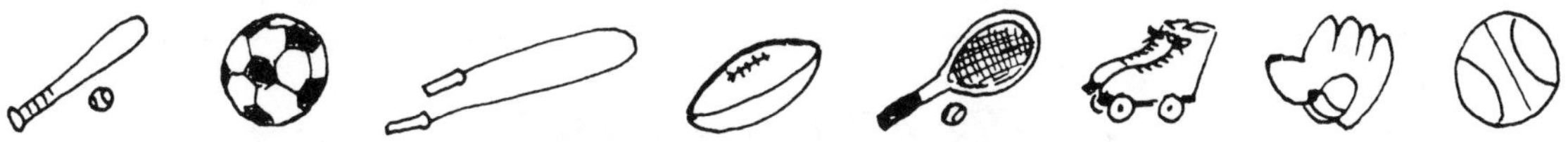

8–6 SHOE SCRAMBLE

Materials:

large box or basket

Directions:

Have the players sit in a large circle on the floor and take off their shoes. Put the shoes in a large box or basket in the middle of the circle and mix them up. For a larger class use more than one box. Have the players listen for your clap then hurry to the box, find their shoes, run back to their spaces and put them on.

8–7 SHOE BOX SLIDE

Materials:

four shoe boxes

Directions:

Chalk a starting line on the floor or playground. Chalk a parallel line about 15 feet away. Divide the players into two teams. Have the teams line up behind the starting line. Put two empty shoe boxes in front of each team. Tell the first players in line to step into the shoe boxes. Tell them to listen for your clap, then slide to the other line, turn around and slide back. Continue until each team returns to the starting line.

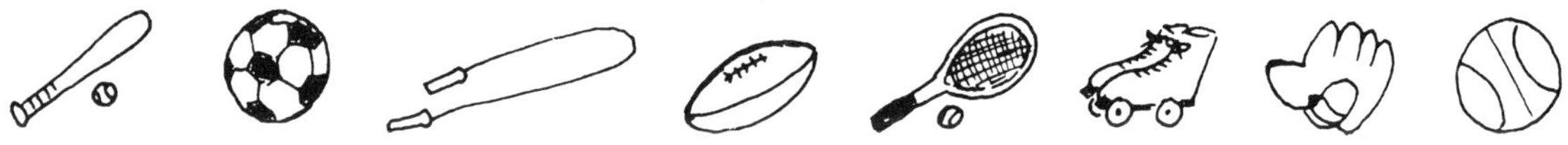

8–8 FEATHER CIRCLE

Materials:

feathers

Directions:

Have the players form several small circles and hold hands. Have one player in each circle throw a feather in the air. The players must blow and keep their feathers in the air without using their hands.

8–9 FOUR PEANUT PICK-UP

Materials:

peanuts
small basket

Directions:

Chalk a long starting line on the floor or playground. Chalk a parallel finish line about 15 feet away. Put a basket in the center of the finish line. Place four peanuts per player, a few feet apart between the two lines. Have the players line up along the starting line. When you clap once the starting player jumps to the peanut closest to him or her, picks it up with one hand, then proceeds to pick up the second peanut with the other hand, etc. When all four peanuts have been picked up the player jumps toward the finish line and tosses the peanuts into the basket and jumps over the finish line. Continue the game until all the players have had a turn.

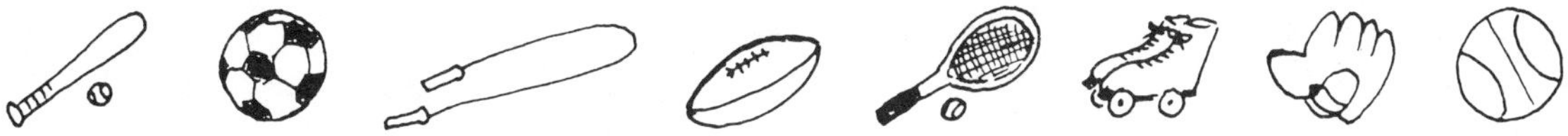

8–10 BELL-RINGER TAG

Materials:

small bell
blindfolds

Directions:

Have the players sit on the floor in a large circle. Blindfold three or four players and have them stand in the middle of the circle. Quietly hand one of the seated players a small bell. Have the bell-ringer stand and move in and out among the blindfolded players while ringing the bell. The blindfolded players try to lightly tag the bell-ringer. The first player who tags the bell-ringer switches places with him or her. Continue the game until all the players around the circle have been active in the game.

8–11 "MEOW, MEOW"

Materials:

cane or yardstick
blindfold

Directions:

Have the players form a large circle. Assign one of the players to be the guesser. The other players are cats. Give the guesser a cane or yardstick and blindfold him or her. Have the guesser stand in the middle of the circle as the cats parade around the circle. When the guesser taps the floor three times with the cane, the cats must stop. The guesser points the cane at one cat. That cat must say, "Meow, meow," slowly and the guesser tries to guess the name of the player. If the guesser gives the right name the cat and guesser change places. If the name is not right the cats continue to march around until the guesser taps the cane again and points to another cat who says, "Meow." The guesser may have three guesses.

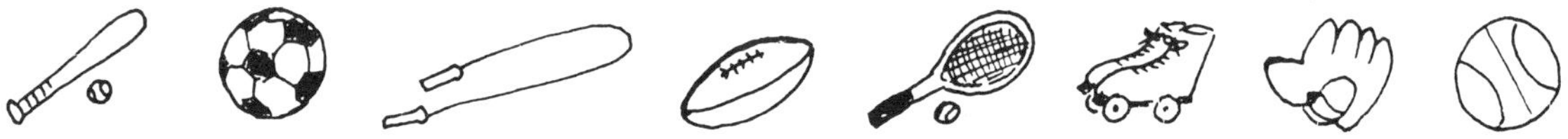

8–12 BALLOON BASKETS

Materials:

balloons
two wastebaskets

Directions:

Chalk a starting line on the floor or playground. Place two wastebaskets about 15 feet away. Divide the players into two teams. Have them line up single file behind the starting line. Give each of the starting players a balloon. Tell them to try and keep their balloons in the air and move to their team's basket. When they hit their balloon into a basket the next player in line will start.

8–13 BALLOON DODGE

Materials:

balloons

Directions:

Divide the players into several small circles. Have a player stand inside each circle. Tell the others to toss a balloon and try to hit the player inside their circle. When a balloon touches a player, he or she must trade places with the player who threw it.

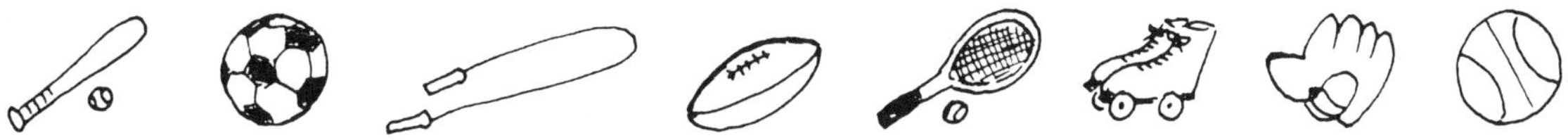

8–14 COLLECT THE COLORS

Materials:

a selection of colored yarn

Directions:

Cut 6″ or 8″ strips of different colored yarn for each player. Scatter the strips around the room. Have the players collect one strip of each color. Vary the game by asking the players to collect a color or colors you request.

8–15 SILLY GOOSE

Have the players stand in a large circle. Assign one person to be the goose. The goose moves around the circle and stops in front of a player. The player must say, "Silly goose, silly goose, silly goose," without laughing. The goose moves to each player in the circle and tries to make them laugh. A player who laughs becomes the silly goose.

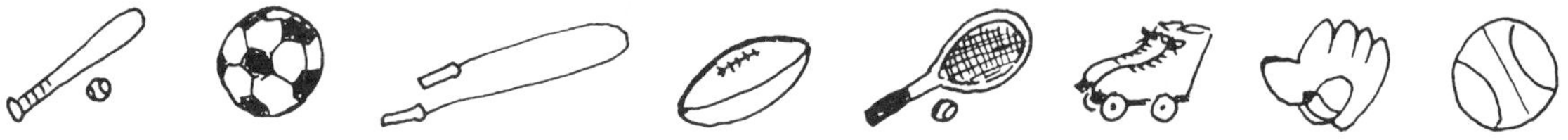

8–16 WHERE IS BOBO?

Assign one player to be IT. Have the other players sit in a large circle around IT. When IT points to one of the players and asks, "Where is Bobo?," the player must answer, "What is Bobo wearing?" IT describes some of the clothing another player is wearing. When the player being described recognizes the description, he or she chases the player who asked, "What is Bobo wearing?" around the circle. The player being chased tries to run back to his or her space without being tagged. If caught, the player becomes IT and the game continues. Make sure everyone has a turn being IT.

8–17 DOT-TO-DOT DASH

Chalk and number 15 or 20 large dots on the floor around the room. Draw a starting line a few feet away from the first dot. Have the players line up single file behind the starting line. Tell them to listen for your hand claps. Explain that one clap means to stand still and two claps mean to move. Proceed, randomly switching between one and two claps. On the first two claps the first player in line runs to dot number one. With the next two claps the player moves to dot number two and the next player in line starts. Continue until all the players have completed the course. Repeat the game having the players jump, skip, crawl or hop around the numbers.

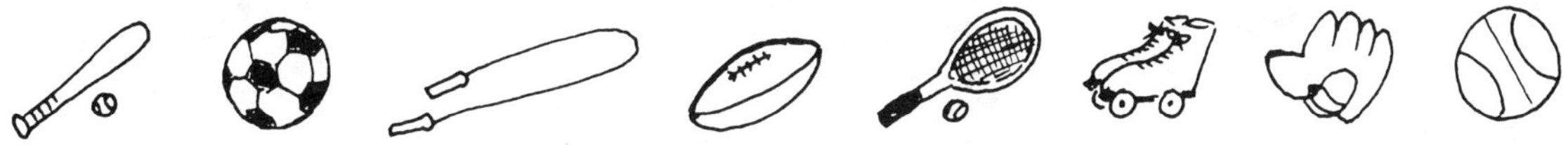

8–18 COUCH POTATOES

Chalk a large circle on the floor or playground. Assign one player to be IT. The other players are couch potatoes who sit around the circle with their eyes closed. Tell IT to move around the inside of the circle chanting:

"Couch potatoes, open your eyes.
Get up and do some exercise!"

The couch potatoes must stand up and exercise inside the circle while IT counts to ten slowly. Continue the game until everyone has had a turn being IT.

8–19 FOLLOW ME, FRIEND

Have the players sit in a large circle. Assign one player to be IT. IT goes up to someone in the circle, takes his or her hand and says, "Follow me, friend, and do as I do." The player chosen follows and does the action IT does. IT may hop, skip, jump, dance, etc. around the circle. Then the follower becomes IT and the two players go up to another player around the circle. The game continues until there are no players left sitting.

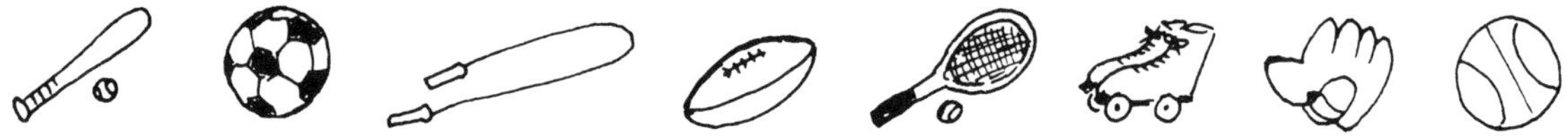

8–20 CAT WANTS A CORNER

Chalk a large square on the floor or playground. Assign one player to be the cat. Four other players stand in one corner each. The cat moves to each corner and says: "Cat wants a corner." The players send him or her to another corner. While the cat is moving towards another corner, the other players try to change places. The cat tries to move into an empty corner. If he or she is successful, the player who left the empty corner becomes the cat.

8–21 RABBIT HOP

Chalk a starting line on the floor or playground. Chalk a parallel line about 12 feet away. Have the players line up along one line. Tell them to put their hands on their knees and jump to the second line. Tell them to turn around and rabbit hop back to the starting line.

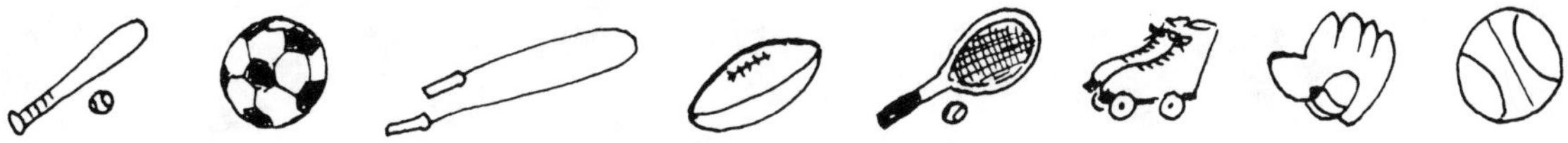

8–22 TURTLE RACE

Chalk a long starting line on the floor or playground. Chalk a parallel line about 20 feet away. Tell the players they are all turtles. Have the turtles line up along the starting line. Tell them to crawl as slowly as they can, without stopping, over the finish line. See who can be the slowest turtle in the race.

8–23 DRIVE ALONG THE LINE

Chalk a long winding line on the floor or playground. Have the students stand in a single file along the line. Tell them to listen for your clap then pretend to drive along the line. After a few minutes, call out, "Turn your cars around." Have the students drive in the other direction.

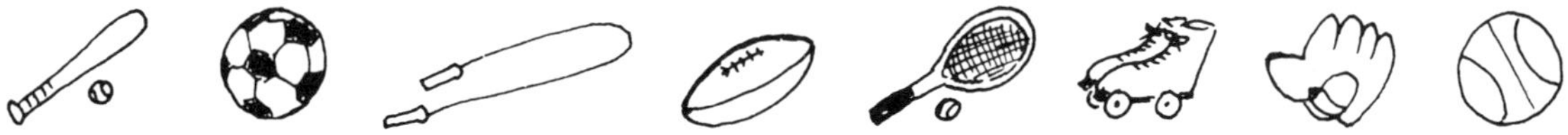

8–24 THE WAVE

Have the students sit in a circle. Assign one student to be the starter. Tell the students to listen for your clap. Have the starter stand quickly and raise his or her arms overhead. The starter sits down quickly and the one to his right stands quickly and raises his or her arms overhead, then sits down. Continue the wave and have the students try to move the wave fast and slow.

8–25 TAKE THE TRAIN

Have the players form a single line. Tell them to put their left hands on the shoulders of the person ahead of them. Have them hold their right arms at waist level and move them in a circular motion. Have the engine pull the players down the tracks and lead everyone in making train noises. Give everyone a turn being the engine.

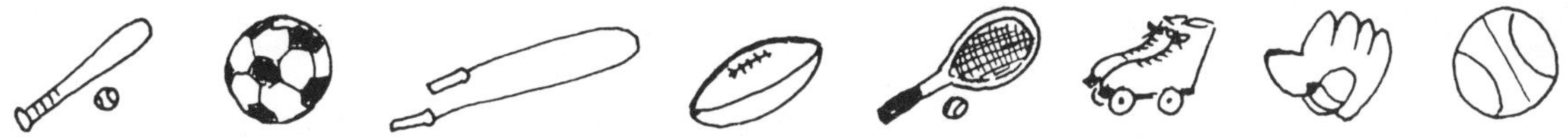

8–26 PONIES GO A-GALLOPING

Have the students stand in a large circle. Read the poem aloud and tell the students to gallop around like ponies in the same direction.

Ponies go a-galloping, a galloping.
Ponies go a-galloping all around the track.

When the ponies have galloped for awhile have them change directions by reading the next verse aloud:

Ponies change directions, directions.
Ponies change directions and gallop back.

8–27 TRAVEL TO THE CITY

Tell the players to listen to the rhythms you clap. Have them listen to the chant and move as it tells them:

Travel to the city
And drive, drive along.
Drive to the city
When you hear this song.

Vary the pace with fast, slow and medium beats. Change the words of the chant at various times to skip, march, run, hop, gallop, strut, crawl, jump, swim, prance, fly, dance, etc. The players return to their seats to rest when you chant this verse:

Travel to the country
And drive, drive home.
Drive home to the country
And do not roam.

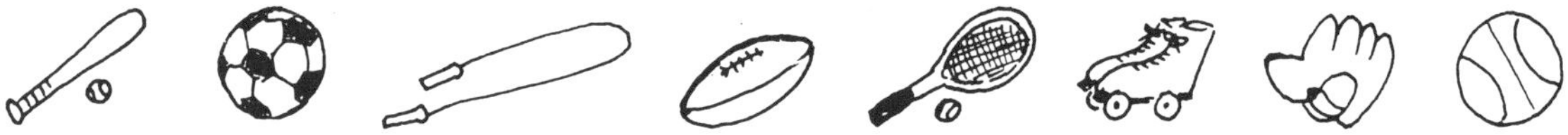

8–28 DRAGON DANCERS

Have the students line up single file with their hands on the shoulders of the person in front of them. Have the students follow as the head of the dragon leads them around the room with up and down and zigzag motions. Continue the dance until everyone has had a turn being the head of the dragon.

Variation: Dragon Chase:

Have the players line up single file with their hands on the shoulders of the person in front of them. Have the dragon head lead the players around the room. The dragon head tries to catch the tail of the dragon. When he or she touches the tail lightly the two change places and the tail becomes the head of the dragon.

8–29 RUN, MICE, RUN

Chalk a long line on the playground. Print "Mouse Hole" behind the line. Chalk a parallel line about 30 feet away. Assign one player to be the cat. All the other players are mice. The mice line up along the mouse hole and the cat stands behind the other line. The mice move slowly towards the cat. When they are in front of the cat they say, "What time is it, Mr. Cat?" The cat says, "Five o'clock," or some other time. When the cat answers, "Midnight," the mice scatter and try to run back to their mouse hole before the cat catches them. The cat lightly tags as many mice as he or she can. The mice who are tagged must stay with the cat and help catch more mice the next time.

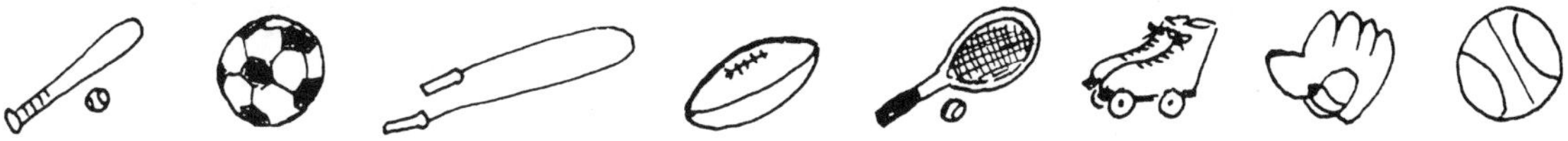

8–30 ROBOTS

Assign one player to be the winder. Have the other players line up single file. The winder moves along the line winding an imaginary key on each player's back. The players then move around like robots. When a robot feels like he or she is winding down it must head slowly back to the winder to be rewound. Have the robots parade around the room single file. Continue the game until everyone has had a turn being the winder.

8–31 RIBBON DANCERS

Materials:

crepe paper in various colors
scissors
record player or cassette player
records or cassettes

Directions:

Cut several colors of crepe paper streamers for each student. Have the students hold two or three different colors in each hand. Play the music for the students. Tell them to move to the music with their streamers. Encourage them to move the streamers in circles, numbers, squares, triangles, waves, etc. Tell them to run with the wind and hold their streamers over their heads.

8–32 HULA HAPPY ME

Materials:

record player or cassette player
record or cassette of Hawaiian music
luau lunch

Directions:

Read the movement poem aloud and have the students sway to the music. Then enjoy a delicious luau lunch.

Hula, hula hips
Swaying to and fro.
Hula, hula hands
Telling tales they know.
Hula, hula feet,
Dancing by the sea
Moving to the music,
Hula happy me.

LUAU LUNCH

You'll need:

an assortment of fresh, canned, frozen or packaged tropical fruits
napkins
sharp knife
small paper plates

Wash all fresh fruits thoroughly. Carefully cut into slices. Arrange on paper plates. Serve with fruit juice or sugar-free drink.

8–33 DANCE TO THE DRUMMER

Materials:

a small drum

Directions:

Have the students form a large circle. Assign one person to be the drummer. The other students are dancers. Tell the drummer to beat the drum slowly at first as the dancers move around the circle to the beat. The drummer may stop the music at any moment and the dancers must freeze. Tell the drummer to vary the beat from slow to fast. Continue until all the students have had a turn being the drummer.

8–34 DANCE, SHADOW

On a sunny day your class can shadow dance outdoors. They can also enjoy shadow dancing indoors.

Materials:

a strong light

Directions:

Shine a strong light on a wall several feet away. Have the students stand between the light and the wall and watch their shadows dance as they do the motions to the poem. Read the poem aloud:

Come, shadow,
Dance, shadow,
Sun's coming out.
Swirl, shadow,
Leap, shadow,
Swing all about.
Sway, shadow,
Turn, shadow,
Time now to end.
Bow, shadow,
Sit, shadow,
Rest, shadow friend.

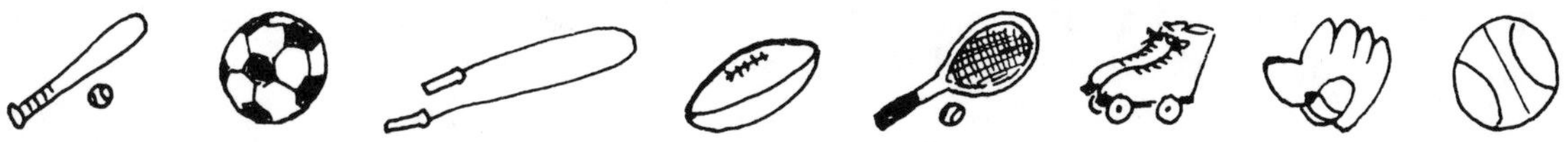

8–35 ICE SKATING

Materials:

record player or cassette player

a record or cassette of "The Skater's Waltz," or other waltzes

Directions:

Chalk a large rectangle on the floor. Chalk a large figure 8 at each end of it. Have the students take off their shoes and put on pretend ice skates. Play a waltz and have the skaters glide around in the ice skating rink. Have the skaters take turns alone or with a partner.

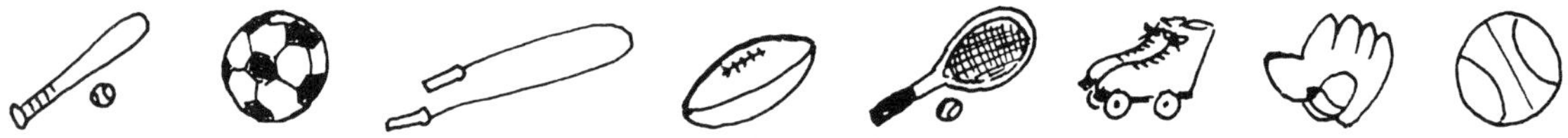

8–36 TOWER TOSS

Materials:

chalk or tape

cardboard box or wooden box

small ball

beanbag

several empty plastic or cardboard containers

Directions:

Chalk or tape four lines on the floor a few feet apart. Put an upside down box several feet away from the lines. Stack the containers on top of the box.

Ask the students to line up at the line closest to the box. Have each student take a turn throwing a ball at the containers to see how many they can knock down. Restack the containers each time.

When each student has had a turn at the first line, repeat the game at the second line using a beanbag, a ball at the third line and a beanbag at the fourth line.

8–37 TAP DANCERS

Materials:

record or cassette player
record or cassette of tap dance music

Directions:

Ask the students to put on imaginary tap shoes. Play a record or cassette of tap dance music and have the students tap dance on a hard surface.

Suggestions for recording or cassette:

– *Music for Tap and Jazz Class,* Kimbo Educational, 1987

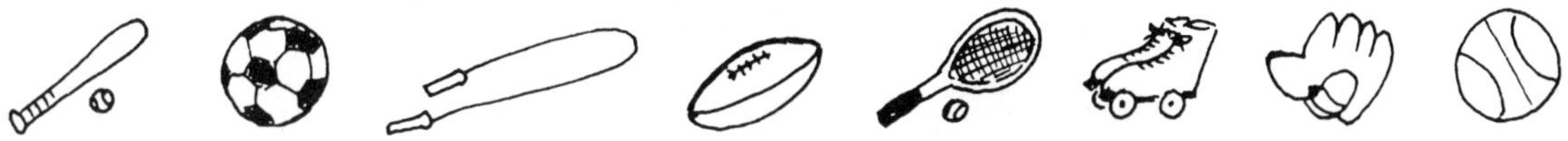

8–38 BALLET DANCERS

Materials:

record or cassette player
record or cassette of Tchaikovsky's *Swan Lake, Sleeping Beauty,* or *The Nutcracker*

Directions:

Have the students put on imaginary ballet shoes. Play a record or cassette of ballet music and let the students move like graceful ballet dancers.

8–39 TUNNEL CRAWL

Divide the players into two teams. Have each team form a single row and stand with their legs apart. Tell the players to listen for your clap then the last player in each line crawls through. Have them continue playing until everyone has had two turns crawling through the tunnel.

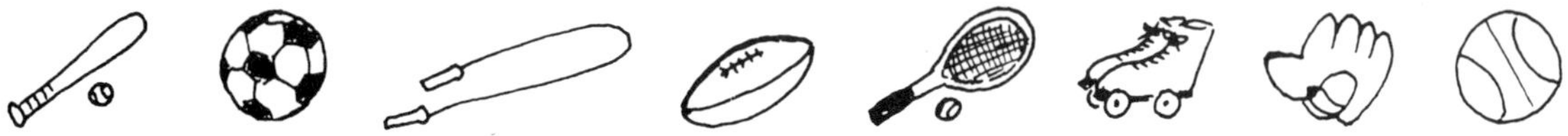

8–40 JUMP, JUMP, HANDSHAKE

Have the players form two rows on opposite sides of the room, facing each other. Tell them to listen for your clap then the first player in each line jumps across to the other team and shakes hands with all the other players in line. Then he or she jumps to the back of the row. Continue until every player has had a turn jumping and shaking hands with the opposite team.

8–41 TOUCH THE GROUND

Chalk a large circle on the floor or playground. Have the players form a circle around the line and count off from one to ten. Tell the ones to stand in the center of the circle and think of some part of the body they want the other players to touch on the ground. Tell them to chant:

Come into the circle and turn around
Then touch your *left knee on the ground.

When all the ones have stepped inside the circle and followed directions, they return to the line. The twos, threes, etc., take their turns in the center. The game continues until all the numbers have had a turn chanting.

*Some suggestions are elbows, toes, feet, thumbs, ears, cheeks, fingers, arms, shoulders, heels, wrists, foreheads, etc.

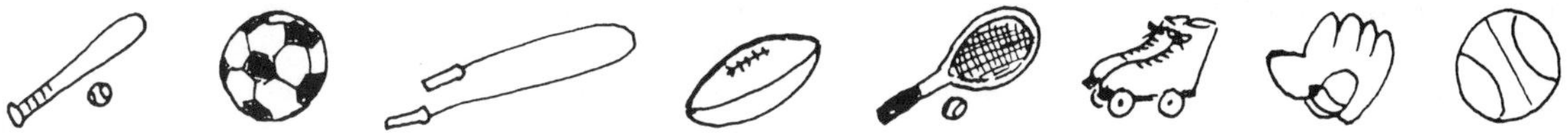

8–42 PAPER BAG BALL

Materials:

large brown paper grocery bags

Directions:

Have each student crumple a large brown paper grocery bag into a ball shape. Show them how to toss the bag ball into the air and hit it with the palms of their hands. Ask the students to see how long they can keep the ball in the air without it touching the ground.

8–43 HOPSTICKS HOME!

Materials:

5 chopsticks

Directions:

Chalk a starting line on the floor or playground. Divide the class into groups of five. Have the first five players stand in line behind the starting line. Tell the other students to sit on the floor several feet away.

Lay 5 chopsticks parallel to the starting line and about 15 inches apart on the floor in front of the players. Tell the first person in line to listen for your clap then try to hop over the sticks without touching them. After hopping over the last stick in the row the player hops around, picks up the closest stick and hops back to the starting place calling out, "Hopsticks home!"

When the four remaining players have returned home ask them to sit down. Lay the five chopsticks down again and begin the game with a new group of players. Continue until each group has had a turn.

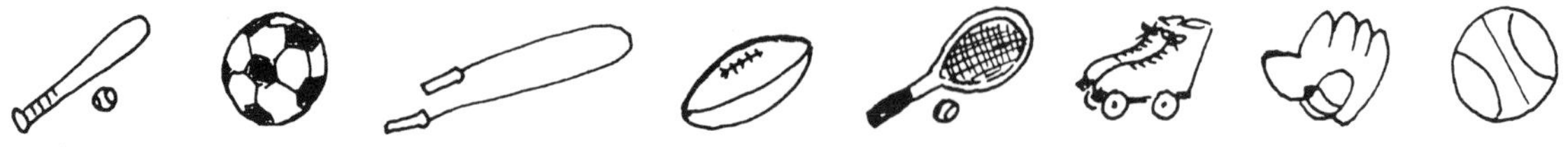

8–44 HIGH BRIDGE, LOW BRIDGE

Assign a few students to be boats and have them form a line a few feet away from the other students.

Have the other students form two lines facing each other, making sure everyone has a partner. Tell the partners to hold hands and raise their arms high to form a bridge.

Have the bridge partners chant the poem as the boats move in a line under the bridge several times:

High bridge, high bridge,
Boats go moving by
Sailing on the river
When the bridge is high.

Tell the bridge partners to listen for your clap then chant:

Low bridge, low bridge,
Boats must wait to go
Sailing on the river
When the bridge is low.

The boats must wait in line until you clap again and the bridge partners repeat the first verse. Let everyone have a turn being a boat.

RESOURCE LIST

The following books, records, cassettes, and videotapes can be used to supplement the activities and reinforce the health concepts presented in HEALTHY, HAPPY, AND FIT! If you are unable to find these resources in your area, most can be ordered from:

Children's Book & Music Center
2500 Santa Monica Blvd.
Santa Monica, CA 90404
Telephone: (213) 829–0215 (in California)
(800) 443–1856 (outside California)

An asterisk (*) before a listing denotes a record, cassette, or videotape.

Nutrition:

BALIAN, LORNA. *Garden for a Groundhog* (Abingdon Press, Nashville TN, 1986)

DRAGONWAGON, CRESCENT. *Alligator Arrived with Apples* (Macmillan, New York, 1987)

EHLERT, LOIS. *Growing Vegetable Soup* (Harcourt Brace Jovanovich, San Diego CA, 1987)

FUJIKAWA, GYO. *Let's Grow a Garden* (Putnam Publishing, New York, 1978)

KANDOIAN, ELLEN. *Is Anybody Up?* (G. P. Putnam's Sons, New York, 1989)

KRAUSS, RUTH. *The Carrot Seed* (Harper & Row, New York, 1945)

MODESITT, JEANNE. *Vegetable Soup* (Macmillan, New York, 1988)

Recipes:

Alpha-Bakery published by Gold Medal Flour (order from General Mills, Inc., P. O. Box 1113, Minneapolis MN 55440)

The Berkeley Co-op Food Book edited by Helen Black (Bull Publishing Co., Berkeley CA, 1980)

FLINDERS, CAROL; ROBERTSON, LAUREL; and RUPPENTHAL, BRIAN. *Laurel's Kitchen* (Ten Speed Press, Berkeley CA, 1986)

Food for Little People (City of Berkeley Department of Public Health, Berkeley Unified School District, Berkeley CA, 1973)

JENKINS, KAREN S. *Kinder Krunchies* (distributed by Discovery Toys, Pleasant Hill CA 94523)

Health Habits:

ANDERSON, LENA. *Bunny Bath* (Farrar, Strauss and Giroux, New York, 1986)

BERENSTAIN, STAN and JAN. *The Berenstain Bears Visit the Dentist* (Random House, New York, 1981)

BERENSTAIN, STAN and JAN. *The Berenstain Bears Go to the Doctor* (Random House, New York, 1981)

BERRY, JOY WILT. *What To Do When Your Mom or Dad Says . . . Go To Bed!* (Childrens Press, Chicago, 1983)

CARLSTROM, NANCY WHITE. *Jesse Bear, What Will You Wear?* (Macmillan, New York, 1986)

CIVARDI, ANNE and CARTWRIGHT, STEPHEN. *Going to the Dentist* (EDC Publishing, Tulsa OK, 1987)

CIVARDI, ANNE and CARTWRIGHT, STEPHEN. *Going to the Doctor* (EDC Publishing, Tulsa OK, 1989)

CIVARDI, ANNE and CARTWRIGHT, STEPHEN. *Going to the Hospital* (EDC Publishing, Tulsa OK, 1987)

KUKLIN, SUSAN. *When I See My Doctor* (Bradbury Press, New York, 1988)

LINN, MARGOT. *A Trip to the Dentist* (Harper & Row, New York, 1988)

LINN, MARGOT. *A Trip to the Doctor* (Harper & Row, New York, 1988)

NEWFIELD, MARCIA. *Where Did You Put Your Sleep?* (Macmillan, New York, 1983)

O'BRIEN, ANNE SIBLEY. *It Hurts!* (Henry Holt & Co., New York, 1986)

ROCKWELL, HARLOW. *My Dentist* (Greenwillow, New York, 1975)

ROCKWELL, HARLOW. *My Doctor* (Macmillan, New York, 1973)

ROGERS, FRED. *Going to the Doctor* (G. P. Putnam's Sons, New York, 1986)

WESTCOTT, NADINE BERNARD. *Getting Up* (Little, Brown & Co., New York, 1987)

Feelings and Self-Esteem:

ALIKI. *Feelings* (Greenwillow, New York, 1984)

ALIKI. *The Two of Them* (Greenwillow, New York, 1979)

ALIKI. *We Are Best Friends* (Greenwillow, New York, 1982)

BRANDENBERG, FRANZ. *I Wish I Was Sick, Too!* (Greenwillow, New York, 1976)

HAVILL, JUANITA. *Jamaica's Find* (Houghton Mifflin, Boston, 1986)

HAVILL, JUANITA. *Jamaica Tag-Along* (Houghton Mifflin, Boston, 1989)

HUBBARD, WOODLEIGH. *C is for Curious, The A, B, C of Feelings* (Chronicle Books, San Francisco CA, 1990)

LEONARD, MARCIA. *How I Feel: Silly* (Bantam, New York, 1988)

MCPHAIL, DAVID. *Sisters* (Harcourt Brace Jovanovich, San Diego CA, 1984)

MORRIS, ANN. *Loving* (Lothrop, Lee & Shepard, New York, 1990)

*PALMER, HAP. *Getting to Know Myself* (Educational Activities, Freeport NY 11520)

PRESTON, EDNA MITCHELL. *The Temper Tantrum Book* (Penguin, New York, 1976)

*RAFFI. *Everything Grows* (A & M Records, 1987)

*ROGERS, FRED. *Mister Rogers: A Place of Our Own* (Mister Rogers Neighborhood Records, 1984)

SHARMAT, MARJORIE WEINMAN. *A Big Fat Enormous Lie* (E. P. Dutton, New York, 1978)

Safety:

BERENSTAIN, STAN and JAN. *The Bike Lesson* (Random House, New York, 1964)

BERENSTAIN, STAN and JAN. *The Berenstain Bears Learn About Strangers* (Random House, New York, 1985)

CHLAD, DOROTHY. *Safety Town* series (Children's Press, Chicago, 1982–1989)

GIRARD, LINDA WALVOORD. *Who Is A Stranger and What Should I Do?* (Albert Whitman, Niles IL, 1985)

*PALMER, HAP. *Learning Basic Skills Through Music: Health and Safety* (Educational Activities, Freeport NY 11520)

VOGEL, CAROLE G. and GOLDNER, KATHRYN A. *The Dangers of Strangers* (Dillon Press, Minneapolis MN 55415, 1983)

Exercise:

BERSHAD, CAROL and BERNICK, DEBORAH. *Bodyworks: The Kids' Guide to Food and Physical Fitness* (Random House, New York, 1976) This book also covers nutrition.

**Get a Good Start: Aerobic Fitness Activities for Young Children* (Kimbo Educational, Long Branch NJ 07740)

ISENBERG, BARBARA and JAFFE, MARJORIE. *Albert the Running Bear's Exercise Book* (Clarion Books, New York, 1984)

**Mousercise* (Disneyland Records, 1982)

TRIER, CAROLA S. *Exercise: What It Is, What It Does* (Greenwillow, New York, 1982)

**Kids in Motion* (Youngheart Records, CBS/Fox, 1987)

The following books are for adults:

HUTH, HOLLY YOUNG. *Counterplay: Focusing Your Child's Energy* (Simon & Schuster, New York, 1984)

PRUDDEN, BONNIE. *How to Keep Your Family Fit and Healthy* (Reader's Digest Press, New York, 1975)

Substance Abuse Prevention:

GARNER, ALAN. *It's O. K. to Say No to Drugs!* (Tom Doherty Associates, New York 10010, 1987)

SEXIAS, JUDITH S. *Alcohol: What It Is, What It Does* (Greenwillow, New York, 1977)

The following books are for adults:

CURRAN, DOLORES. *Traits of a Healthy Family* (Harper & Row, San Francisco, 1983)

Growing Up Drug Free: A Parent's Guide to Prevention (order from U. S. Department of Education, Washington, D. C. by calling 1-800-624-0100)

WILMES, DAVID J. *Parenting for Prevention* (Johnson Institute Books, Minneapolis, 1988)

Games and Dances:

BLEY, EDGAR S. *The Best Singing Games for Children of All Ages* (Sterling Publishing Co., New York, 1981)

*JENKINS, ELLA. *And One and Two* (Folkways Records, Princeton NJ, 1971)

MILLEN, NINA. *Children's Games from Many Lands* (Friendship Press, New York, 1969)

**Music for Tap and Jazz Class* (Kimbo Educational, Long Branch NJ 07740, 1987)

NELSON, ESTHER L. *Dancing Games for Children of All Ages* (Sterling Publishing Co., New York, 1974)

ROCKWELL, ANNE. *Games (& How to Play Them)* (Thomas Y. Crowell, New York, 1983)

SERNAQUE, VIVIENNE. *Classic Children's Games* (Dell Publishing, New York, 1988)

**Sharon, Lois & Bram's Elephant Show Record* (Elephant Records, Toronto, Canada, 1986)

*STEWART, GEORGIANA LICCIONE. *Folk Dance Fun* (Kimbo Educational, Long Branch NJ 07740, 1984)

*STEWART, GEORGIANA LICCIONE. *Fun Activities for Perceptual Motor Skills* (Kimbo Educational, Long Branch NJ 07740, 1976)

WISWELL, PHIL. *Kids' Games* (Doubleday, New York, 1987)

*ZEITLIN, PATTY and BERMAN, MARCIA. *Rainy Day Dances, Rainy Day Songs* (Educational Activities, Freeport NY 11520, 1975)